"Orthorexia, although largely _____, is a prevalent issue among food bloggers who constantly compare and compete to see who can have the best, the healthiest, the most virtuous diet. And while veganism is a wonderfully fulfilling and healthy lifestyle when it's done correctly, many young and impressionable girls are citing veganism as an excuse to dangerously restrict their food intake in a quest to purify their bodies. Jordan learned the hard way that even a vegan diet can be unhealthy when it's not a *balanced* vegan diet. Her speaking out will hopefully inspire others to question their own food rules and restore balance to their lives."

—Katie Higgins, author of *Chocolate-Covered Katie* and founder of chocolatecoveredkatie.com

"Jordan's story mirrors that of what so many of us women go through: shame, self-doubt, and a hungry search for well-being. I hope women read her story and find the inspiration and nourishment she discovered in learning to listen to her own body."

—Alexandra Jamieson, C.H.H.C., C.A.P.P., author of *Women, Food, and Desire*

"I'm constantly impressed by Jordan's bravery and ceaseless commitment to growth, no matter how difficult. She is an inspiration to anyone who wants to change their lives, and living proof that one can do it with joy, grace, and compassion."

—Kelsey Miller, senior features writer at Refinery29.com and author of *Big Girl: How I Gave Up Dieting and Got a Life*

"For anyone who has struggled with an eating disorder, or knows someone who has, *Breaking Vegan* is a must-read. Jordan's honest and brave portrayal of what it is like to struggle with every bite will help many girls, boys, women, and men to recover from their struggle. She helps to let you know you are not alone, and that recovery and a happy life with food are possible."

—Jamie Graber, founder of Gingersnap's Organic cafe

"*Breaking Vegan* is incredibly honest, and Jordan's decision to fight for her personal happiness is very inspirational. It's a book that all young people need to read, regardless of their dietary choices."

—Max Goldberg, founder of LivingMaxwell.com and The Pressed Juice Directory

". . . an extremely well-written book that will change your relationship with food and teach you how to care for your body and feel your best. I am so ecstatic this story is being told and applaud Jordan for her transparency and courage to share her experience."

—Annie Lawless, co-creator of SUJA Juice and coauthor of *The Suja Juice Solution*

". . . a transparent peek inside of Jordan's personal life and an inspirational bible for intuitive living, with the scripture being, 'there's no one size fits all—and that's allll gooood.'"

—Emily Nolan, founder of mykindoflife.com

"Younger's brave journey toward self-acceptance will resonate with anyone who's craved control over their diet or image. This candid memoir is a fascinating account of orthorexia, an eating disorder that takes healthy eating to dangerous extremes."

—Alexandra Orlov, writer at DailyBurn.com

BREAKING
VEGAN

ONE WOMAN'S JOURNEY FROM
VEGANISM, EXTREME DIETING,
AND **ORTHOREXIA** TO A
MORE BALANCED LIFE

JORDAN YOUNGER

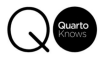

Quarto is the authority on a wide range of topics.

Quarto educates, entertains and enriches the lives of our readers—enthusiasts and lovers of hands-on living.

www.QuartoKnows.com

First published in the United States of America in 2016 by
Fair Winds Press, an imprint of
Quarto Publishing Group USA Inc.
100 Cummings Center
Suite 406-L
Beverly, Massachusetts 01915-6101
Telephone: (978) 282-9590
Fax: (978) 283-2742
QuartoKnows.com
Visit our blogs at QuartoKnows.com

20 19 18 17 16   1 2 3 4 5

ISBN: 978-1-59233-700-2

Digital edition published in 2016
eISBN: 978-1-62788-789-2

Library of Congress Cataloging-in-Publication Data available

Cover and book design by Kathie Alexander

Page layout by Megan Jones Design

Photography by Tynan Daniels Photography, except pages 12, 19, 22, 25, 35, 56, 74, 76, 77, 159, and 167, courtesy of Jordan Younger.

Printed and bound in China

From the publisher: The information in this book is for educational purposes only. It is not intended to replace the advice of a physician or medical practitioner. Please see your health care provider before beginning any new health program.

dedication

For *each* and *every* one of my blog readers.
My love for all of you is unreal.

And for the two people who have made me everything I am—
my *mom* and *dad*. There are no words to express my love and gratitude.

disclaimer

This is not a book bashing veganism. This is not a book saying veganism
causes eating disorders. This is a book that captures my personal journey
through veganism, how I took it too far, and how many of us with extreme
personalities may be capable of doing the same.

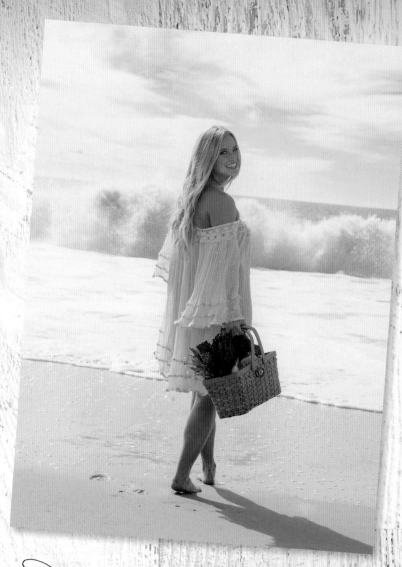

For you

"For anyone who has ever gotten lost in an extreme and felt that there was no way out; For anyone who has controlled an aspect of his or her life through food, exercise, or any outer source rather than dealing with a problem head-on; You are not alone. Balance is within reach."

CONTENTS

FOREWORD

BY STEVEN BRATMAN, M.D., M.P.H

Can eating healthy food become an eating disorder?

The idea sounds patently ridiculous. We live in a society where high fructose corn syrup infests the supermarket shelves, antibiotics and other chemicals pile up in the food chain, and obesity starts in childhood. Any intelligent person interested in health would naturally want to find a better diet than the one on offer.

Nonetheless, *some* people who are devoted to healthy eating develop an eating disorder in relation to that focus. This disorder is called *orthorexia nervosa*, which may be defined informally as a focus on healthy food that involves other emotional factors and becomes dysfunctional, even dangerous. Consider this analogy: It is indisputably healthy to maintain normal weight and avoid obesity. However, in pursuit of this goal, and in combination with psychological factors, *some* people develop anorexia nervosa. A similar process can happen with healthy food.

To be clear, choosing healthy food does not equate to orthorexia. Quite the contrary. People can adhere to just about any theory of healthy eating without having an eating disorder (with the caveat that their diet must provide adequate nutrients). For example, veganism in itself is *not* an eating disorder. However, some vegans do become orthorexic.

The Origin of the Term

When I coined the term "orthorexia nervosa" in the 1990s, I didn't realize I was naming an eating disorder. I was a practitioner of alternative medicine at the time, and although a proponent of a healthy diet, I thought a few of my patients took it too far. I remember one in particular who began every visit by asking, "Doctor, what food should I cut out?" I had seen her dozens of times over a two-year period and eventually came to believe that the last thing she needed was to cut any more foods out of her diet. In my opinion, she would benefit most from doing exactly the opposite: relax the grip of her mind, ease her self-imposed food restrictions, and live a little.

But I understood where she was coming from. More than a decade earlier, I had been obsessed with dietary perfection myself, first as a follower of macrobiotics and then as a raw foods vegan. Because of this personal experience, I knew how difficult it would be for her to hear the advice I wanted to give. To advise her to lighten up on her diet was tantamount to asking her to embark on a life of crime, as if I were to say, "Go and commit a little larceny! It will be good for you." She saw a healthy diet as pure virtue. How can one lighten up on a virtue?

After some consideration, I decided to stand her virtue on its head by calling it a disease. I consulted a Greek scholar and coined the term *orthorexia nervosa*. The word is formed in analogy to anorexia nervosa, but using *ortho*, meaning "right," to indicate an obsession with eating the right foods.

From then on, whenever this patient would ask me what food she should cut out, I would say, "We need to work on your orthorexia." This made her laugh, and ultimately it helped her loosen the lifestyle corset. She moved from extremism to moderation.

Later, I published a funny article on the subject and then a humorous book with a bad cover color scheme and the badly chosen title *Health Food Junkies*. I didn't take my own idea too seriously. I just wanted to get a few overly obsessed health foodists to take a look at themselves. It was only after the publication of the book that I began to realize I had tapped into something bigger: I learned that there are people who die of orthorexia.

That was a shock. I understood that people could make themselves crazy trying to maintain a healthy diet, but not that they could go so far as to injure themselves via malnutrition. Unlike people with anorexia, individuals with this type of severe orthorexia don't think they're too fat; they think they're impure and need to cleanse. These are distinctly different motivations.

Because the concept of orthorexia was still little known at this time, eating disorder specialists often misunderstood such patients. They would say to them, "You think you are too fat." But that is not what it feels like to be orthorexic. This misunderstanding led to treatment failure, with occasionally tragic results. (Note: Some people, such as Jordan, seem to combine features of both anorexia and orthorexia, but when orthorexia predominates it must be addressed as such for treatment to succeed.)

Even when orthorexia is not fatal, it can commandeer a person's life. Eating disorders have that power.

The Power of a Word

Since the early 2000s, serious academic study of orthorexia has blossomed. Organizations such as the International Federation of Eating Disorder Dietitians and the National Eating Disorders Association began to discuss the concept at meetings and in their published literature. In 2014, Thomas R. Dunn, Ph.D., of the University of Northern Colorado, published a formal article in the journal *Psychosomatics* on a case of orthorexia and proposed formal diagnostic criteria. A somewhat different set of criteria was proposed by Jessica Setnick, M.S., R.D., C.E.D.R.D., in *The Eating Disorders Clinical Pocket Guide, 2nd edition*. The authors of *The Diagnostic and Statistical Manual of Mental Disorders* (*DSM*), the American Psychiatric Association's classification and diagnostic tool, began discussing adding it to their next revision.

Perhaps most important of all, young women such as Jordan Younger have now begun to say to themselves, "I want to eat healthy food, but I don't want to be orthorexic."

Naming is powerful. When it comes to food, we need all the power we can get because food can make you crazy. It hits you in the heart and goes straight to your self-esteem. It taps into all that is lonely and empty and needy and promises to fill that emptiness. It triggers dark places. It can tie up your mind in knots so intricate and strong that even the search for healthiness can become unhealthy.

Against this, the word *orthorexia* serves as a signifier. It is a kind of mental signpost to indicate a limit, a boundary not to go beyond even in search of healthy diet. And, if you've already gone beyond, it can help you find your way back.

This is what happened for Jordan. After achieving fame as a proponent of veganism, she came to understand that she had orthorexia. Since then, she has been live-blogging her awakening. This is a brave and powerful act.

DO YOU HAVE ORTHOREXIA?

When Jordan's public self-discovery led to increased media awareness of orthorexia, I contacted her and learned about her history. Her journey does not describe every person's path. It is personal to her demographic, her childhood, and herself. But if you have orthorexia, you will recognize your own processes here.

Do you wonder whether you have orthorexia? For instance, do you turn to healthy food for happiness, for meaning?

Eating the perfect diet might make you less likely to get cancer, and it could prevent bloating and give you more energy—*but it won't make you happy*. Using food as primary refuge is a form of spiritual materialism. You are filling the space that longs for love with mere *stuff*. To quote Jordan, "I was entering into a relationship with veganism . . . veganism became my boyfriend, my best friend, and my confidant."

Does your healthy diet make you feel important? "The strict diet helped me feel extraordinary when I was very fearful of being ordinary."

Does eating a healthy diet make you feel in control? Do you have to keep upping the ante to get the same kick? "[Veganism] triggered a desire within me to be more and more extreme, more and more pure, and to achieve more and more nutritional perfection to the point where no foods were safe."

Do you use diet to ward off anxiety, not just about health, but about everything? Has the idea of healthy food become a kind of brain parasite, taking over your life, ceasing to serve you and instead making you its slave?

If you recognize yourself in any of this, read this book. If it resonates, consider consulting an eating disorders specialist who understands orthorexia. It may change your life. It may even save it.

Steven Bratman, M.D., M.P.H., *began his career as an organic farmer in upstate New York in the late 1970s. After attending medical school, he practiced alternative medicine, including acupuncture, herbal medicine, and dietary therapy. In the late 1990s, he directed a research project evaluating and summarizing all published scientific evidence on alternative medicine methods. He coined the term "orthorexia" in a 1997 article in* Yoga Journal. *He is the author and editor of numerous articles and books, including the* Natural Health Bible *and* Health Food Junkies. *Currently, he practices preventive/occupational medicine in the San Francisco Bay Area.*

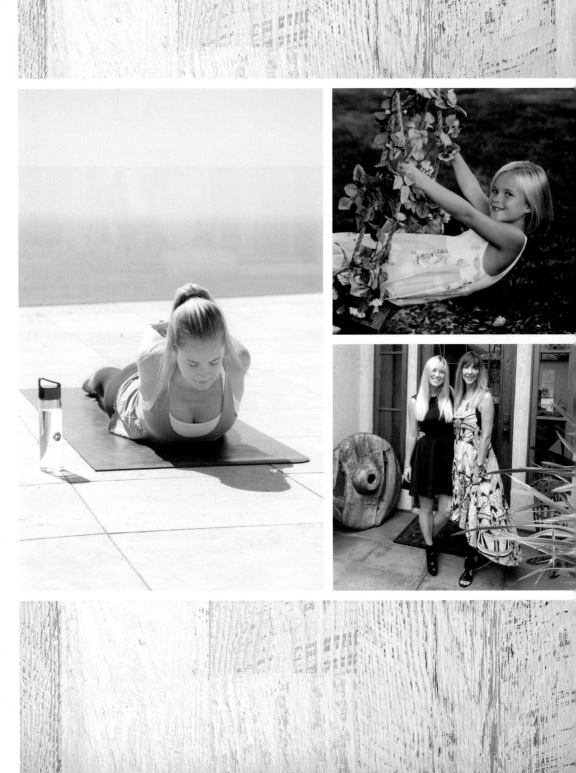

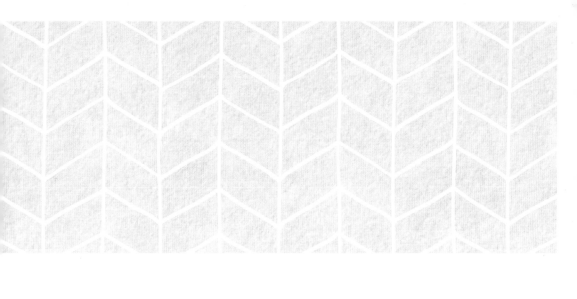

MY STORY

PART 1

Veganism, Orthorexia
& Everything in Between

Let's Get Real

Want me to be really real here? This book has been extremely hard to write. It's been a challenge for both my mind and my psyche. Since it's such an important story for me to share, I've often felt like there could be no way to properly convey it in its entirety. As long as I can remember, I've never experienced any type of writer's block or any issues getting my thoughts down on paper. When I was in fourth grade, for example, I wrote a hyper-detailed ninety-six-page story on the Monterey Bay Aquarium in California, complete with an eclectic cast of talking sea creatures. Tell me to write a brand-new blog post on a different topic every day? Done. Write freelance articles up the wazoo? Hell yes. Sit down and write a book about something deeply personal that I am extremely passionate about? *Uhhh, here's the funny thing about that . . .*

Long projects intimidate me to no end, especially when they are based on something I care about very much. Hard as they may be, however, there isn't anything I care more about than sharing this story with you. That's not because I'm dying to discuss the depths of my soul for the first time or seeking some kind of sympathy about my story that will make me feel better about my eating issues as a whole. And it's certainly not because I think anyone's journey toward balance can be tidied up with a little red bow by simply getting it down on paper.

It's important to me to share this story because when I was in the midst of my eating disorder, I felt so, so alone. I felt alone in a way that was terrifying, and I felt like I was going to have obsessions and compulsions around food forever.

I want to share this story with you because whether you've suffered from an eating disorder or not, whether you've ever slapped a label on your diet, or whether you've even heard of the term *orthorexia*, I think you can relate to the challenges that come along with that delicate search for balance, both in food and in life.

When I started recovering from my eating disorder and transitioning from veganism, I quickly learned that I had been applying my all-or-nothing personality to absolutely everything in my life. My relationships were all-or-nothing, my work was all-or-nothing, and my thirty-day juice cleanses and intense avoidance of non-plant-based foods were all-or-nothing.

And so, being an all-or-nothing kind of girl, sitting down to write a full-length memoir is *daunting*. I write spur-of-the-moment, off-the-cuff blog posts every morning! My words and stances and opinions get to evolve with the ebb and flow of my everyday life and recovery process. But what I've had to remember in writing this book is that I am writing about a specific time in my life. I am writing about developing an eating disorder and falling prey to the stronghold it took over my personality and my livelihood. I'm writing about my powerful love affair with veganism and my descent into a full-blown obsession with "pure" foods and achieving the so-called perfect body and the perfect state of health.

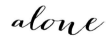

alone

"WHEN I WAS IN THE MIDST OF MY EATING DISORDER, I FELT SO, SO ALONE. I FELT ALONE IN A WAY THAT WAS TERRIFYING, AND I FELT LIKE I WAS GOING TO HAVE OBSESSIONS AND COMPULSIONS AROUND FOOD FOREVER."

Coming out of veganism, I have yo-yoed up and down a lot. I have flip-flopped with dietary choices, with weight, with dedication to exercise, and with dedication to recovery. It is *hard* to strike a balance after emerging from a severe case of extremes where I disconnected every fiber of my being from the ability to listen to my body. But I've done it, and I'm here. I've lived through it, and I want to help you do the same.

The truth is, we are all in this together. Instead of comparing ourselves and tearing each other down, we should be empowering one another to fall in love with our bodies and with our lives—*to find balance*. But before we can make any big life changes, we must first examine our back story—and we all have one. Eating disorders, as with all life challenges, don't just material-ize without a logical reason.

My reason was . . . well, I had many. From a lifelong sensitive tummy, to an extremely intense dedication to veganism, to rapid weight loss, to soul-crushing family problems, to becoming a successful vegan food blog-ger in a short amount of time, I went through it all, up and down, and my eating disorder quickly developed from minor to full-fledged.

Even though this story was sometimes hard for me to get out, now it's all on paper and I am so happy to share it with you. Yes, you. Thank you for picking it up. It's not just an eating disorder story, but also a glimpse into my life during a transformational, albeit rocky—I won't deny it—period of time. A real-life character sketch, if you will. It's reality TV on paper! I hope you find some comfort in my story, some inspiration, some laughs, and maybe (just maybe!) you will find some thought-provoking moments that motivate you to think about where in your life you would like to stretch, grow, and evolve.

Let's get started, shall we?

From my heart to yours,

Jordan

1

DIARIES OF AN EXTREME-A-HOLIC

I have to begin by telling you that my food intake and I have an extremely complicated origin story. Think lifelong stomach sensitivities that have resulted in pain, bloating, nausea, and ceaseless complaints that made the people around me kind of, sort of want to kill me. Anything with grease, oil, dairy, sugar, wheat, and the occasional unpredictable ingredient would leave my stomach reeling and making some of the craziest noises you've ever heard. If you ask my parents, they will tell you that it's pretty much been this way ever since I sprang from the womb.

As a result of my extreme tummy sensitivity, the precedent was set early on that when I ate well and avoided the foods that drove my stomach crazy, I was praised and complimented for doing so. Alternately, when I gave in and ate what other people around me were eating, I was immediately reminded that I had done something terribly wrong. And hello, I was a kid! Anyone remember the ever-present allure of pizza, ice cream, and chocolaty birthday cupcakes? The Standard American Diet wasn't necessarily easy to avoid as a '90s kid—nor is it to this day!

Essentially, I correlated eating foods that made me feel sick with feeling like I had failed or done something wrong, and I associated avoiding them with unyielding self-control and pride-worthy willpower. I don't know if that association added to my propensity toward an all-or-nothing personality or if I would have turned out that way regardless. I'm willing to bet it's a little bit of both.

I distinctly remember being eleven years old, complete with rainbow-colored braces, SpongeBob shoelaces, and pigtail braids, standing in the doorway of my family's pantry stocked with sugary cereals and bags of chips and declaring to myself that I would "never, ever, as long as I lived touch any of *that* food again." I made the impulsive decision based on the calmness in my stomach that I only experienced when I felt totally empty. Even though avoiding junk and processed food seemed doable in theory, I was too young to carry it out in a way that would be sustainable long-term.

It was around then that I developed a routine where I would restrict for days, sometimes even weeks at a time, and then cave whenever a certain event or situation with food came up—or more often, when I just got too hungry. The willpower of restriction made me feel like a rock star, while the caving, on the other hand, always made me feel pretty helpless. But the routine in itself was consistent even in its inconsistency.

At that young age, eating healthfully wasn't on any of my friends' radars, and I certainly didn't understand the science and details behind nutrient-dense foods versus processed. All I knew was that eating well made me feel good and that extreme dieting was really ridiculously hard to maintain for long periods of time.

willpower

"ESSENTIALLY, I CORRELATED EATING FOODS THAT MADE ME FEEL SICK WITH FEELING LIKE I HAD FAILED OR DONE SOMETHING WRONG, AND I ASSOCIATED AVOIDING THEM WITH UNYIELDING SELF-CONTROL AND PRIDE-WORTHY WILLPOWER."

The Childhood Years

The first time I correlated food with weight gain and the absence of food with weight loss was when I was about nine years old. I was at my cousin's birthday party, and I was proudly sporting a star-studded one-piece bathing suit from The Gap. I was playing with my boy cousins and my nephew, jumping into the pool, running in the grass, and trying not to get tagged to be "it." While we were playing around, my mom was talking to my older sister. I couldn't make out all the words, but the only thing I heard loud and clear was my sister saying, "No, I don't think she's gotten chubby. I think she's just growing."

I stopped running and listened more closely. Now I was intrigued. There was no way they could be talking about me, I thought. But after assessing the situation for a second, I knew they had to be. They were looking my way, subtly but surely, and there was no other *she* they could be talking about—I was the only young girl in our family who was out by the pool. And geez, maybe I *had* gotten a little chubby, I thought. I mean, had I? I knew I weighed more than my best friend, 9 pounds (4.1 kg) to be exact, because we'd weighed each other for fun in her mom's bathroom just a few days prior; but I figured that was normal because she was stick skinny and that's how her body was built. Everyone knew she was really skinny. Was I really that much bigger than her?

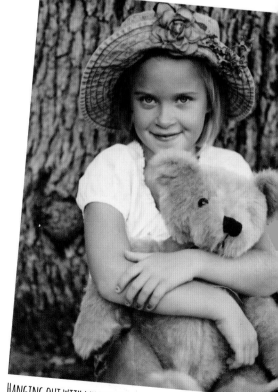

I looked down at myself in my dripping, star-spangled one-piece. Maybe I was looking a little round? It was hard to tell because I wasn't exactly sure who to compare myself to. I was kind of in the middle size range of all my friends from what I could tell. I had lost a lot

HANGING OUT WITH MY TEDDY BEAR IN THE MID-90s

of weight the year before, when I had whooping cough and pneumonia and threw up everything I ate for three months straight, and I knew at that time my mom and my doctors talked about how serious the weight loss was for someone my age. I knew it because I heard them talk about it, but I didn't feel it or notice it. Weight was *far* from my mind. I just wanted to be healthy so I could go to school with my friends and show off my new inhaler!

So maybe I had just gained it all back? Maybe they were talking about it because I finally looked healthy again after being sick, I thought. But then why would they use the word *chubby*? I tried to find comfort in the fact that my sister apparently disagreed about my chubbiness, but the words still stung. When everyone had hot dogs and hamburgers for dinner that night, I had trouble enjoying them, and I wondered if maybe by eating like everyone else I was doing something wrong.

It wasn't exactly a mental turning point, because I still ate like a regular kid for years to come, but it was definitely the beginning of a new awareness. It was the understanding that other people were looking at me, they were seeing my body for what it was, for better or for worse, and somehow it made me feel like they were assessing my self-control. If they were impressed with what they saw, perhaps they would be impressed by my willpower and my ability to eat well and exercise portion control. They would see an active, sun-kissed, physically fit me whose body didn't need to be overanalyzed.

eating

"IT WASN'T EXACTLY A MENTAL TURNING POINT, BECAUSE I STILL ATE LIKE A REGULAR KID FOR YEARS TO COME, BUT IT WAS DEFINITELY THE BEGINNING OF A NEW AWARENESS."

Alternately, if what they saw concerned them in any way, I would be mortified. It was bad enough that my stomach writhed in pain after I ate just about anything, but learning at that age that food *also* affected the way I looked and how people looked at me was such a tough concept to wrap my head around. I didn't understand why or how people could enjoy junk food in a carefree way if they knew it could make them "chubby," or worse, overweight.

I was too young to understand what it meant to avoid unhealthy foods completely, especially in a world where every special occasion was accompanied by a smattering of hearty foods and decadent desserts, but I was definitely intrigued enough to consider how I might go about eliminating them one day. I felt like if anyone could do it, I could. When I set my mind to something, I made it happen, just like the times I wrote novel-length fiction for a project with a page limit of fifteen or read hundreds upon hundreds of books and logged their summaries into my fifth-grade teacher's Reading Competition notebook, far exceeding the required amount. I'd had a desperate, longing *need* to be the winner—the one who read the most, the one who was praised.

I guess you could say I had a bit of a competitive nature, but I displayed it in funny ways. It mostly came out in competition with *myself*. I was the kind of kid who took the "don't step on a crack, or you'll break your mother's back" game *very* seriously, and from age five to this very day, I have a weird superstition about stepping on the blue and white handicapped parking spot symbol. In fact, in my recent days of recovering from extremes and trying to be more lax, I have stepped on the symbol a few times here and there to show myself it wouldn't kill me. It still gives me an uncomfortable wave of anxiety I have only begun to learn how to deal with.

Competing with myself grew into something else when I got older, something that connected food and willpower and body image and exercise and control—something that could be easily managed by taking rigorous yoga classes every day, eating maniacally well, and making a huge deal about my diet to whoever would listen whenever tummy-friendly food was not readily available. I went in and out of phases like this, as the most extreme of us tend to do. There were weeks when I didn't touch anything that was not a fruit, a vegetable, a rice cake, or an egg white and weeks when I swore to myself I would eat a scoop of ice cream every single day after school because I was young and active and hardworking and stressed out and I freaking deserved it.

The Teenage Years

By the time I was in high school, my relationship with food started to sprout new layers and grow a little more tumultuous. Once I experienced my first heartbreak, food became a bit of an outlet. And it wasn't just a regular heartbreak. The boy I was in love with, blissfully and innocently and beautifully connected to, blossomed from my best friend to my boyfriend (with a few bumps along the way), and we dated from the age of fifteen onward. Tommy was the light of my life. Just thinking about him, I would buzz through the school days with basically two hearts for eyes and then go home and rush through my homework to hang out or instant message with him. He was my confidant and my first taste of what it was like to *know* someone I hadn't grown up with at my tiny little pre-K through twelfth-grade school. He was new and different, and I was sure he was the kindest individual I had ever known.

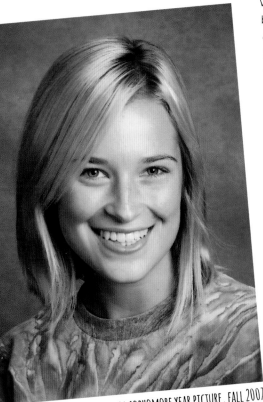

MY HIGH SCHOOL SOPHOMORE YEAR PICTURE, FALL 2007 —TRYING TO BE A HIPPIE IN MY TIE-DYE

When we were sixteen, Tommy started dabbling in the drug scene. First it seemed kind of normal, the same as what a lot of other teenage guys were doing, but as time went on, it became more troubling. He was trying dangerous things that terrified me, and even worse, he was depressed. He wasn't happy with himself or with anything he was doing. Some days when we were together, he wouldn't speak at all. It made me sick to my stomach, and naturally, I obsessed over it. I wanted nothing more in the universe than to make him better.

If we broke up once, we broke up a hundred times, because no matter how many times one of us ended it, the breakup would never stick. I was too worried about him, he felt too bad when I felt even worse about everything, and damnit—were we in love. In December of our junior year of high school, Tommy tried to kill himself. Thankfully he was able to get help before the worst could happen, but upon getting his suicide letter and thinking he was dead, I went berserk.

It was a majorly emotional time of pain, hysteria, worry, and fear that it might happen again. It was an event that changed me, as no doubt it changed everyone who was close to him, in more ways than one. Whenever I am asked if there was a defining moment in my adolescence that separated childhood from adulthood, that is clearly and definitively my answer. I was shattered, and I was hell-bent on making sure Tommy would never get back to that level of emotional vulnerability again. While he dealt with his problems in his own way, I turned to food, and the avoidance of it, for comfort.

When I starved myself, I felt a semblance of control and had a way to express to others outwardly what was happening with me on the inside. I lived for the days when I would arrive at school and one of my friends would say, "Whoa, *you* look skinny!" and I detested the days when I ate too much and felt like my life, and my body, had derailed because of it.

On top of it all, one of the side effects of Tommy's depression was that he had no appetite. When I was with him, all I wanted him to do was eat. I saw him withering away in front of me, and I knew that proper food and nourishment would help him feel more whole. Around then, food took on a whole new meaning for me: healing. Food symbolized health. And even if my mental state didn't feel healthy because I was so worried about what was going on with him, I felt like if I could just *eat well* and get him to do the same, there would be power in it for both of us.

To achieve that level of perfection and control, I cut a whole lot of foods out of my diet. I stopped eating red meat, went gluten-free, and scaled way back on my portion sizes. I lost a noticeable amount of weight and very much enjoyed being able to control any challenges that came my way by restricting my food intake.

I didn't think of it as skipping meals or as not eating enough. I felt like I was just fueling my body with less and less food because that's what it needed to thrive and to feel its best. At the same time, I started doing a lot of reading on processed foods and how they affect the body. I also started doing a lot of yoga. My growing interest in yoga opened up a whole new world in terms of spirituality, health, and the connections between my mind and body. I am so extremely thankful for finding yoga at such a young age because when you read the chapters to come, you'll see that in order to stay afloat, I needed some kind of grounding force in my life.

I had no idea at the time that what I was doing, even at the age of sixteen, was using food to control my emotions and also to control how others perceived me. If I was the lean, fit girl who got attention and recognition for being knowledgeable about healthy food and fitness, I felt like I was on top of the world. When I let my nutrition slip, gained weight, or felt bloated and bogged down by stomach pain, I felt like my outer self didn't reflect my inner passion for health, so in turn, I felt like I was doing something wrong.

Without realizing it, I was using this cycle as a way to classify myself as successful or unsuccessful by way of food. I associated the feeling of starvation with being in control and making healthy choices. When my stomach was empty, I had no stomach pain. When I had no stomach pain, I felt that I had room for more energy. When I had more energy, I felt happier, healthier, and more excited about life and pursuing the things I was passionate about.

It felt good, but even at that point, it felt frighteningly unsustainable.

emotions

"I HAD NO IDEA AT THE TIME THAT WHAT I WAS DOING, EVEN AT THE AGE OF SIXTEEN, WAS USING FOOD TO CONTROL MY EMOTIONS AND ALSO TO CONTROL HOW OTHERS PERCEIVED ME."

The College Days

Fast-forward to college a couple of years later. Now a seasoned yogi and a typical eighteen-year-old chick who thinks she has the whole world figured out, I didn't worry much about the way I looked. I knew I was fit from my daily (often twice-daily) yoga practice and my relatively strong avoidance of unhealthy foods, but right away I realized that the social scene of college was a whole new ballgame. Being the super-social (read: always extreme) person I am, I wasn't about to miss out on anything that seemed like a good time. Party on a Monday night? I was there. Rager on a Saturday followed by a Sunday day party (*darty*, if you will) with loads of alcohol and sugary mixers? Count me in. All-nighters in the library with chocolate chip cookies as big as my face and icy mochas saturated in chocolate sauce? Hell to the yeah.

Inevitably, my previous control over my health started to lose its significance. Hanging out with my friends was my priority, and even though I chose yogurt and granola for breakfast over buttery, syrup-dripping pancakes and I mostly ordered salads instead of the pizza my friends ate late at night, I still knew I was not doing my *best* in the health department. I don't exaggerate when I say that a typical night out consisted of downing eight shots of vodka followed by a 3 a.m. rendezvous with microwaved grits topped with melted cheese or extra-salty pretzels and an extra-large tub of peanut butter. It wasn't an issue of control or lack of control, it was simply my way of letting go of restrictions and living life without giving food a second thought.

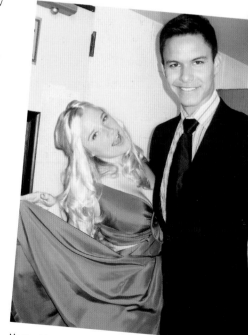

I wasn't eating differently from anyone else I spent time with, but that was part of the problem. I was moving further away from the Jordan I'd once been, who prioritized health and valued a night in reading a good book just as much as a wild night out in Hollywood. During those early college years, I ignored my desire for creative adventures and for being different and

ME AND MY FRIEND JORDAN DORSO IN 2010 DURING OUR FIRST YEAR OF COLLEGE replaced it by pretty much forcing myself to be what I believed normal was supposed to look like.

And even though letting go of some of the things I knew about myself to be a part of the crowd was part of the problem in the overall picture of my eating disorder, at the time, it was exactly what I needed. I will forever admire my younger self for letting loose, abandoning my food rules, and enjoying living every bit of the first few years of college. Just a couple of years later when I was in the midst of my eating disorder, I looked back on that girl and wondered where on earth she'd found the courage to so consistently live in the moment.

All throughout college I told myself that once I graduated, I would make my way back to the super-health-conscious version of myself with a vengeance. I made elaborate plans in my head for my postgrad life, where I planned to get my health, my rockin' bod, and my balanced lifestyle back in order.

And that, my friends, is exactly what I did—and then some. I don't want to scare you off too soon, but now that you have a bit of background about my crazy stomach problems and extreme personality, let's dive on in.

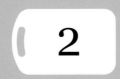

2

MY VEGAN LOVE AFFAIR

There is simply no other way to put it than to say that on a very basic level, I fell head over heels in love with plant-based veganism. The diet and lifestyle allured me from a very young age, and I began working toward living fully plant-based before most people my age had even heard of the term vegetarian. I cut out red meat and pork when I was fourteen in an effort to be more environmentally friendly and also in a desperate attempt to avoid foods that made my stomach feel like crap.

As you know, most food and my tumultuous tummy had made up their minds to be total enemies, so finding a sense of calm by way of fruits and veggies basically made me want to scream *Glory, Hallelujah!* to the plant-based gods. Before I started eating plants in abundance, the foods I ate and my stomach typically dueled it out and left my insides feeling like they had just been through a nasty game of cat's cradle with scissors.

In the beginning, learning about veganism was a harmless interest with innocent intentions. But, like most love affairs, my relationship with the lifestyle took on many forms. There was the schoolgirl-crush phase where I admired it from afar and tried to learn as much about it as I could so I could one day be a part of it—be *worthy* of being a part of it. Then there was the newlywed phase, in which I was ecstatic to be not only a full-fledged plant-based vegan, but a *thriving* full-fledged plant-based vegan. "I'm good at this!" "People come to me to learn more about this diet and lifestyle!" "I'm part of the *club*." "I created the goddamn club." "Veganism and me go way back." "We're buds." "We are in love."

And that's how I am with everything. I test the waters for a little bit, and if it's a match, then boom! I'm all in. If it's not, then I'm over it as fast as it began. I do it with diets, I do it with creative projects, I do it with people, I most certainly do it with exercise, and obviously, I do it with career moves. It's a tendency of us extreme humans: We are all in, or we are all out. And with veganism, I was all in.

After the newlywed phase, there came the "V, we are solidifying this match before we get sick of each other" stage in which I created my vegan food blog and Instagram account. By this point, we had been through quite a bit together. We had traveled together, we had displayed our unwavering dedication to one another at beachside restaurants in Cabo and in gourmet French restaurants in New York City, we had tried several juice cleanses together, and we had purchased extravagant kitchen appliances that never should have seen the light of my bank account's day.

Then, of course, as with all things that are born out of obsession and extremism, veganism and I hit a rocky patch. That's what the majority of this book is about. But before then, we had our glory days. And even though it makes me cringe to think about how rigidly tied to the vegan label I was while I was living it like there was no tomorrow, I know that I initially discovered veganism because I was searching for something more in life. Somehow and in some way, the vegan diet brought that "something" to me. It gave me the feeling of wholeness I was craving so deeply and so desperately that I didn't even know I needed it until I had it.

obsession

"THEN, OF COURSE, AS WITH ALL THINGS THAT ARE BORN OUT OF OBSESSION AND EXTREMISM, VEGANISM AND I HIT A ROCKY PATCH. THAT'S WHAT THE MAJORITY OF THIS BOOK IS ABOUT. BUT BEFORE THEN, WE HAD OUR GLORY DAYS."

I found veganism when I was twenty-two years old. I was a senior in college, and I was scared shitless about what the future might hold. I was sick and tired of the sorority lifestyle, partying hard, staying up until 3 a.m., bingeing on packaged nachos, and waking up at noon to chug a beer upside down. Okay, I know that sounds a little extreme, but I think by now you've gathered that I have a tendency toward extremes. It was suggested to me by people I was close to (including but not limited to my loving yet brutally honest therapist) that maybe it was time to explore "other sides" of myself even though I was still in college—a.k.a. quit your sorority, move out of the house you share with six other girls, focus on things you love like writing and yoga, and stop letting the anxiety and pressure of your social life and relationships take over your brain.

While I wholeheartedly agreed with each of those sentiments, I wasn't quite ready to do that. Essentially, I wasn't ready to be *different* from everyone else I spent so much time with. All my friends seemed to enjoy our regular college lifestyle, and at the end of the day, they appeared totally happy and fulfilled. And because I am still close with many of them, I can attest to the fact that they were and *are* happy and fulfilled. And since that is the case, why was I so tortured by, ummm, let's see here . . . everything?

I mean, I was a happy person. I had good friends, a loving family, did well in school, was generally happy with my body, and felt passionate about the things I was doing in life (school, my English major, sorority, interning at *LA Yoga* magazine, and teaching yoga in my university's gym), but I also felt really freaking depressed. And not depressed in the "I don't want to get out of bed" kind of way, but more in the "I *want* to get out of bed but don't know what the hell I want to do with myself today" kind of way. And also in the "I'm not sure if anyone else in the effing world feels the way I do" kind of way.

I dreamed of a life where I felt a little (or a lot) more in control. I spent hours daydreaming about moving to New York after graduation and writing a novel about the intricate interactions between people and their lovers, sipping on a cappuccino with my hair twisted into a side braid, and animatedly discussing the musings of the universe with people who totally got me. At the core of it, what I was visualizing was a Jordan who was confident enough to do what she loves and not only say screw being different, but believe that being different actually rocks.

In a funny yet totally understandable way, veganism catapulted me into the realm of being "different" from everyone else I knew, and it also gave me some of the tools I needed to feel secure in those differences. I was used to being not much like a lot of my friends. (News flash: I now realize we are all very different and that's what makes our friendships cool and interesting and ridiculously worthwhile.) But even so, I had never really had something to call my *own*, unless you count my massively problematic insomnia or my propensity toward writing 150-page fictional stories in a 48-hour period . . . then no, I really didn't.

The Breakup Diet

I dove into the vegan lifestyle after a pretty soul-crushing breakup in December of my senior year of college. I won't go into too much detail, but let's just say a lot of alcohol was involved, some cheating and some lying on one end, and some absolute shock, betrayal, and terror about what on earth to do next on my end.

It wasn't until that day and the weeks and months that followed it that I understood what it was like to lose your appetite because of pure devastation. I went into fight-or-flight mode, where food wasn't even a fleeting thought. When I did take the time to sit down and eat, I couldn't stomach more than a few bites. A normal plate of food looked monstrous and impossible to dent, so slowly but surely I began to shed major poundage.

And to be honest, I kind of liked it. Who doesn't like losing weight after a breakup? I knew it wasn't healthy to lose it so quickly and it wasn't necessarily sustainable, but I felt powerful and in control as my dwindling frame portrayed the intense emotions I felt on the inside by reflecting them to people who weren't in my body. And, lo and behold, the sneaky and annoying stomach problems I'd dealt with all my life were finally at bay. Without any foods that bothered my tummy going into my system, I caught a glimpse of what it was like to experience a calm and content stomach— *What a concept.* I sort of knew it would be hard to keep up my newfound routine without long-term starving myself (something I never set out to do), but I was hooked on feeling good and was determined to make it last in any way possible.

After about a month and a half of this "breakup diet," in which it would not be abnormal for me to eat only half of an English muffin, a scoop of almond butter, a spoonful of cottage cheese, and a slice or two of raw ahi tuna *in a day*, I set out on a five-day plant-based cleanse with my mom to ring in the New Year. As I said, I had been intrigued by veganism for quite some time, but never had I executed the diet properly in the past. In college, I had attempted a vegan diet by subsisting on no more than tomatoes, avocado, and lemon juice for weeks at a time, but up until then that was my biggest foray into veganism.

This time around things were different. The plant-based cleanse we embarked on included two juices, one smoothie, and two solid food meals per day. The solid food meals were made of fruits, veggies, and nuts, and we were left to our own devices to create them each day. The cleanse company dropped off the liquids each morning, and throughout the day, my mom and I made elaborate, colorful, fruit-filled salads. At night, we baked veggies, playing around with which ones tasted best together, and drizzled them with fresh lime juice and balsamic vinegar to bring out their natural flavors. Spending so much time cooking, creating, and enjoying food from the earth was exhilarating for me, especially after having hardly eaten anything since the breakup.

cleanse

"THE PLANT-BASED CLEANSE WE EMBARKED ON INCLUDED TWO JUICES, ONE SMOOTHIE, AND TWO SOLID FOOD MEALS PER DAY. THE SOLID FOOD MEALS WERE MADE OF FRUITS, VEGGIES, AND NUTS, AND WE WERE LEFT TO OUR OWN DEVICES TO CREATE THEM EACH DAY."

What were my thoughts on the cleanse after the first few days of eating that way? Utter glory! I felt incredible fueling my body with fruits and veggies. I was eating so much more food than I had been during my appetite-suppressed breakup period, but I felt lighter than ever with energy to live my life and get back into my daily workout routine. The water weight my body had been desperately holding on to totally dropped off, and even my skin felt like it was glowing. My parents and the people close to me noticed the quick change and very much encouraged me to keep it up.

And thus the love affair began. It didn't take a whole lot to convince me that eating a nutrient-dense diet of predominantly organic produce high in vitamins and minerals was a wonderful way to fuel my sensitive body. Food from the earth is easy on our digestive systems, and it powers our minds and bodies so we can perform at our highest level. I became a walking, talking billboard for eating a whole heck of a lot of plants, and in those early days, the benefits I experienced far outweighed any difficulty I felt about the lifestyle being "different" from what I was used to.

During that time, the nutrients and enzymes from the fruits and vegetables flooded my body and gave me an energy that felt a bit like awakening from a deep, tummy-pain-induced sleep. And now that I was eating normal amounts again, I felt stronger and ready to move beyond my breakup and create a new, bolder, redefined version of myself that was itching to be released into the world.

During that week, I decided I wasn't going to go back to my previous way of eating, and I knew what that meant. It meant I was adopting a vegan diet, and I was finally doing it the *right* way: full of fruits and veggies and nutrient-rich juices and smoothies. I made my newfound diet clear to everyone around me, in hopes that shouting it from the rooftops would help explain the radical shift taking place within me. The problem was, it was all still so new, I made a lot of mistakes in the beginning. Even so, I was determined to make it work—it was the first and only style of eating that didn't rip my stomach apart, and I was not going to let it pass me by.

3

NO ONE PLANS TO DEVELOP AN EATING DISORDER

Right after the initial plant-based cleanse and my decision to start eating vegan, I took a road trip from Sacramento to LA with my best friend Jillian to start our last semester of college. When we stopped to get gas on our way out of town, Jill looked me up and down and said, "Holy shit, Jo! I have never seen you this tiny!" Of course I played it off like I barely knew what she was talking about (*"Who, me?!"*), but inside I was glowing because I knew that my outer frame reflected the mind-body connection I was developing with my plant-based diet.

The drive is six hours long, so midway through we stopped to get something to eat. Jillian got orange chicken and vegetable fried rice from a Chinese takeout place—yes, I'm that creepy friend who remembers people's orders verbatim years later—while I cracked open my leftover butternut squash soup from the cleanse and ate a few big spoonfuls until I felt satisfied. I remember the look on her face that very clearly read, "That's *all* you're going to eat?" and then her many attempts to get me to try a bite of her deep-fried chicken. It was a no-go.

We chatted the drive away about life, the wild New Year's Eve we'd just had in San Francisco, and how panicked I was to run into my now ex-boyfriend once the semester started back up. We were planning to go to a pajama-themed party that evening and decided that when we got back into town, we would go shopping for cute matching pajamas. (Jillian ended up swapping her pajamas with my friend Sarah, pictured with me on page 35, at the party.) I wanted to have some kind of plant-based snack beforehand because the soup barely sustained me for more than an hour, but I didn't have any snacks with me and it made more sense to drive straight to the mall. I told myself it was fine—I could embrace the empty feeling, as I'd done many times before.

But as we shopped, I felt myself getting hungrier and hungrier, to the point where I felt like I could faint at any moment. By the time we picked out the perfect heart-printed boxers and matching white tees and were standing in line to buy them, I told Jillian if we didn't get dinner immediately, I thought I might pass out. We had only one small issue: Neither of us knew of any restaurants where I could order clean vegan food and she could order something non-vegan, or what I started learning from there on out to refer to as "regular" food.

We researched up a storm on our phones and learned that one of our favorite pizza places in Venice Beach also had a farm-fresh seasonal veggie plate. Score! Now the concern was getting there before my stomach chomped away at itself. Jillian kept offering that we go into a Starbucks and grab a snack for me or at least a protein bar, but I was so determined

hunger

"WHAT I WAS EXPERIENCING WASN'T JUST RUN-OF-THE-MILL HUNGER; THIS WAS TWO MONTHS' WORTH OF EXTREME DEPRIVATION AND A WEEK SPENT ON PURELY FRUITS AND VEGGIES WITH NO GRAINS, FATS, OR SUGAR WHATSOEVER. MY BODY WAS RUNNING ON ZERO."

to stick to my cleanse (even though it was over), I wasn't going to stop until we found plain steamed vegetables and/or a piece of fruit.

We went back to the car to drive to the restaurant, and by the grace of God, we made it there before my stomach ate itself and my mind along with it. I knew the service at this particular restaurant was usually quick, so I figured things would be fine once we walked in. But, of course, there was a *long* line, and my hope dwindled yet again. I actually remember thinking that if I could just get to the front of the line, place my order, and get a glass of water, then I could suck on the lemons from the condiments bar until the food came. (Crazy-town, right?)

Alas, there were no lemons to be had, and the fifteen-minute wait was one of the most uncomfortable and agonizing experiences I can recall in my life. What I was experiencing wasn't just run-of-the-mill hunger; this was two months' worth of extreme deprivation and a week spent on purely fruits and veggies with no grains, fats, or sugar whatsoever. My body was running on zero.

Jillian's food came first, and despite the misery of my hunger, I refused to take even the tiniest bite of her pizza to hold myself over. It wasn't even an option in my mind because I was so afraid it would derail all the hard work I had put in to cleanse my system and feel good. When my veggie plate finally came to the table, however, I went to town on the broccoli, brussels sprouts, and leafy greens. I ignored the beans, raisins, and pesto on the plate even though they

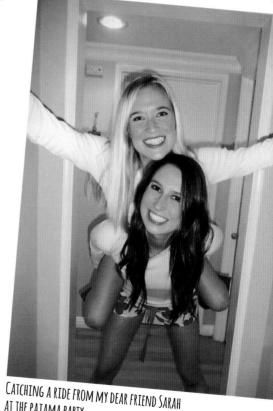

CATCHING A RIDE FROM MY DEAR FRIEND SARAH AT THE PAJAMA PARTY

looked delicious and satisfying because I was trying hard to hold on to the "cleanse" guidelines (fruits, veggies, and nuts only). It was a wonder I had any self-control left because I had reached a level of hunger I didn't know was possible—but I was still learning, I told myself. It was my first week on a plant-based diet, and there was no way I was going to give up that light and energized feeling it gave me.

For the rest of the night, I felt bloated, self-conscious, and, for lack of a better word, *huge*—even though I was most certainly at the lowest weight I had been since I was a preteen. I look back on photos from that night and shudder to think I believed that one meal of pure veggies, of which I ate probably one-quarter, would make me gain back all twenty pounds (9.1 kg) I'd lost. That night is monumental in my eyes because it was the first time I let food totally dictate my mood, my body image, and the amount of fun I had. I avoided alcohol at the party and wanted to go home early because I felt panicked just being around it.

The whole way home, I kept saying to my roommates, "I think I'm a little over house parties," and "We've just done the same thing so many times, it's not really fun anymore." Although my words had an element of truth, my inner food demons were really what kept me from having fun that night, and I knew it. Though I kept my newfound fixation pretty hidden, the amount of time I spent obsessing about it in my mind made up for the lack of talking about it out loud. Even being at that pajama party where people were playing beer pong and making late-night pizza runs made my anxiety spike. Not to mention all I could think about was waking up the next morning and exercising to burn off what I'd eaten for dinner—vegetables.

Taking Control

From that night on, I learned to be ultra-prepared when it came to packing snacks in between my tiny meals, and I also learned that overeating, even of plant-based foods, always led to feelings of guilt and self-loathing. To me, this was another step toward controlling the exact amount of food I put into my body and another brick in the wall when it came to mentally correlating my food intake and my happiness level.

To get right down to it, I was entering into a relationship with veganism. In the beginning stages of the diet, veganism became my boyfriend, my best friend, and my confidant. Instead of letting the pent-up emotion from my actual breakup keep me in a sad, dark place, I poured it into learning about my new lifestyle and "evolving" into a healthier version of myself. I wanted to know everything there was to know about veganism, from the leaders in the lifestyle to the science behind the diet to the restaurants that catered to it. I wrote research papers on veganism, interviewed influential vegans for my journalism classes, and spent countless hours on my computer watching vegan YouTube channels and reading vegan blogs.

To say I was obsessed would be an understatement. And now I see why. The strict diet helped me feel extraordinary when I was very fearful of being ordinary. I was twenty-two and at a huge turning point. A very important and serious relationship in my life had just ended, I was about to graduate college and enter the world as a postgrad, and I was on the verge of moving across the country and living away from California for the first time.

What twenty-two-year-old isn't freaking terrified of what their young adult life has in store for them? I am a dreamer and an idealist. Believe it or not, those are two things I now love about myself, but at the time, they had me terrified that I was chasing a dream that was never going to come true. I was moving to New York to be a fiction writer, for God's sake—that's more or less the equivalent of moving to Los Angeles to become Hollywood's next hot actress. I loved the idea of dreaming big, but I was panicked about whether or not it would work out.

I wanted very much to excel at what I loved and to find great success in doing it, but I was extremely fearful that my MFA endeavors would lead me to nothing more than a desk job that I wasn't passionate about. I knew I had

best friend

"TO GET RIGHT DOWN TO IT, I WAS ENTERING INTO A RELATIONSHIP WITH VEGANISM. IN THE BEGINNING STAGES OF THE DIET, VEGANISM BECAME MY BOYFRIEND, MY BEST FRIEND, AND MY CONFIDANT."

it in me to write the fiction I had been jotting down and dreaming up in my head for years, but I had no idea whether I could carry it out as a career or whether anyone would care.

Veganism was something I could hold on to—something so clear in its principles, there was no way I could fail. Plus, it was just out-of-the-ordinary enough that it gave me an identity when I was so desperately searching for one to latch on to. Even deeper, it was the one way I could maintain the "happy" stomach state I experienced from eating next to nothing . . . except with veganism, I could actually eat fruits and veggies and drink fresh juices *while* maintaining the "benefits" of more or less starving myself.

I will add that I knew all along that veganism wasn't the *only* thing that made me stand out, but at the time, making an extravagant dietary change gave me the extra confidence I needed to go out into the real world with a clearer identity. Veganism encompassed my passion for health and my dedication to go all in with the things I love. Cooking vegan food and coming up with new plant-based recipes served as a creative outlet. It was also a way for me to connect with people and teach them about what I loved without having to continuously immerse myself in things I was no longer very excited about, like alcohol, partying, and the large space both of those had taken up in my social life for the past several years.

No one plans to develop an eating disorder. No one plans to become an addict. No one *wants* to feel the pain and difficulty of going through something hard in order to come out on the other side, but sometimes things just happen, and we have to roll with it. Veganism gave me something to hang on to during a time when I needed unyielding reassurance. Eventually I would find my way toward a more balanced life, but I still had a ways to go before getting there. And before it got better, it got a whole lot worse.

4

SERRATED KNIVES & THE BIRTH OF THE BLONDE VEGAN

I was totally convinced that the years I had spent consuming processed food and drinking toxic beverages like endless shots of vodka chased with ginger ale caused damage that could only be undone by eating fresh, organic, pure, whole food from the earth (yes, all that criteria had to be met) and completely avoiding anything that could potentially harm my body. I very much believed that plant-based veganism was an evolved lifestyle—this awesome, semisecret society that few knew about and even fewer understood, but one that everyone would eventually catch on to and join.

I wasn't preachy about my views on food, and that's mainly because I don't have a preachy nature (thank God). I did, and still do, very much understand that no diet under the sun works perfectly for everyone. That said, I did believe that when practiced correctly, and without preexisting health concerns or serious deficiencies, a plant-based vegan diet *could* suit everyone just fine. I believed that plant-based veganism was the most surefire way to ward off future disease and weight gain. I also got very attached to the idea that the diet was the most sustainable for the earth and kindest toward animals—a cornerstone of veganism that only perpetuated my obsession.

Essentially, following a plant-based diet made me feel like a boss. I didn't necessarily feel like I was better than non-vegans because of my diet, but somewhere inside, I felt like I was doing something pretty damn awesome, through willpower alone.

In those first several months of veganism, I enjoyed every ounce of the lifestyle and didn't have any cravings or desires to eat anything that didn't fall under the vegan umbrella. Substituting unhealthy foods with healthier ones came naturally to me. I loved eating quinoa, lentils, and roasted veggies for dinner and very much preferred the natural flavors of my home-cooked meals to the salty, saucy restaurant food I grew up on.

Cooking plant-based foods became a creative outlet. I loved experimenting in the kitchen and creating new recipes. I adored styling the colorful food on my plate and snapping photos of it. I really got into reading vegan food blogs, and I lusted after the gorgeous photos of smoothies and salad bowls filled to the brim. I followed vegan dessert blogs such as *Chocolate-Covered Katie* and *Oh, Lady Cakes* and silently wondered whether I would ever allow ingredients like brown sugar—or even coconut sugar—to pass my lips again. I thought I might incorporate certain things back into my diet eventually, when I was more used to the vegan lifestyle, but I certainly wasn't there yet.

My "cookies" were made from mashed overripe bananas, oats, almond butter, flaxseed meal, walnuts, and a few all-natural, dairy-free chocolate chips if I was feeling like an extra treat. Even though the cookies were basically bite-size, if I ate two in a day I felt as if I had way overindulged, and then I worked out to the max to make up for it.

cooking

"COOKING PLANT-BASED FOODS BECAME A CREATIVE OUTLET. I LOVED EXPERIMENTING IN THE KITCHEN AND CREATING NEW RECIPES. I ADORED STYLING THE COLORFUL FOOD ON MY PLATE AND SNAPPING PHOTOS OF IT."

Because of my extremely clean diet, I felt the effects of every last gram of food I put into my body. There is something kind of cool about that—and also something a bit alarming. If I indulged in a few bites of a raw dessert made with cacao and coconut oil, I woke up with what felt like an oil hangover and regretted it for hours until it passed through my system. If I ate a few more brussels sprouts than usual or had an extra couple of scoops of quinoa on my plate, I felt a heaviness in my stomach later that night and the next morning. Similarly, if I didn't add a spoonful of almond butter or a bit of flaxseed meal in my smoothie each morning, I felt I didn't have the sustenance to get me through my first few classes. It was a delicate balance in a very food-dependent kind of way.

Becoming so attuned to the relationship between the food I was eating and its effect on my body was a very interesting experience, and in some ways, it was the most addicting part of the lifestyle. My energy and well-being depended so heavily on the balance of vitamins, minerals, and protein that eating became somewhat of a sacred practice. I couldn't go anywhere without planning what I was going to eat and when I was going to eat it, so my once-haphazard, spontaneous routine quickly became more regimented.

I sometimes look back on those early days of veganism and wonder how I became that person. In the beginning, I was vegan because I was listening to my body. Eliminating foods that had always bothered my stomach felt good, and before I started calling myself a vegan, I didn't flip out if there was a smidge of cheese in my salad or if a raw ahi lettuce wrap sounded better than a veggie lettuce wrap. But the moment I realized that the diet I was following fell under the category of plant-based veganism, I ran with it—it was all-or-nothing.

Even though the lifestyle had its challenges, I was elated that my stomach problems had seemingly disappeared. I explained my diet to others by saying, "I've finally eliminated everything that made me feel like crap," versus "I eat plants and only plants," which made me seem and feel less extreme in the beginning. I had fun concocting vegan desserts in the kitchen and modifying my once-beloved chocolate chip cookie and fudgy brownie recipes to overflow with nutrients and health properties. I classified food based on its nutritional benefits (cacao: antioxidant; honey: energy; banana: potassium; prebiotic: energy; etc.). Obviously my prior attachments to store-bought frozen yogurt, corn tortillas, salt-and-vinegar chips, and the intermittent peanut butter cup no longer fit the health-addicted bill.

It's when I started to lose that satisfied and content feeling in my stomach, however, that things started to get trickier. I didn't want to question my vegan diet, but I did question the portion sizes and food combinations I was eating. I started toying around with different veggies and eating more gluten-free grains, and when all else failed and my stomach still hurt, I just reasoned that I needed to keep a tighter hold on my diet. I needed to be as clean and pure as possible, even if it meant eating less than my body desired or needed.

Even though I didn't want to question my veganism, when I was around people who knew me really well, at times I tried to feel the situation out. The first time it happened was on another cross-state drive with Jillian, my last before I moved to New York, while we were once again discussing my sensitive stomach. Outwardly I had been adamant that my vegan diet had cured my stomach problems, but after eating that way for about six months, I was starting to slip into a lull, and I couldn't totally hide it. I felt bloated again and didn't feel like I radiated the super-healthy aesthetic I did when I first started the diet. I didn't want to admit that any part of my vegan diet might be failing me, but Jill, as those few and far between soul-mate friends often do, had the distinct ability to pull the truth out of me.

"I feel like eating fish and eggs *once in a while* might be better for me than having to eat so many fruits and vegetables to feel full all the time . . . I mean, like very rarely, but maybe sometimes," I ended up saying, most definitely avoiding eye contact.

And Jill, being that kind of a friend, said, "That's a great idea. You love sushi; why deprive yourself? If you want to try it, I'll go to sushi with you tonight. I'll even order fish." (She doesn't like sushi. That's a real friend.)

Truth

"I DIDN'T WANT TO ADMIT THAT ANY PART OF MY VEGAN DIET MIGHT BE FAILING ME, BUT JILL, AS THOSE FEW AND FAR BETWEEN SOUL-MATE FRIENDS OFTEN DO, HAD THE DISTINCT ABILITY TO PULL THE TRUTH OUT OF ME."

This may or may not come as a surprise, but we didn't go to sushi that night. I woke up the next day declaring that I had changed my mind about reincorporating fish and eggs into my diet and that my doubt must have come from a moment of exhaustion or hunger. In fact, it was about time for another cleanse—a three-day juice cleanse this time, which would be my first time going more than just one day on liquids alone.

I woke up at the crack of dawn to drive, in the pitch black, to pick up my eighteen juices from a juice bar an hour away. I couldn't risk getting hungry and having to eat a bite of solid food precleanse that morning, so the odd hours had to be done. Who cared if I was going to spend my morning sitting in rush hour traffic on the way back into Los Angeles? I would have my green juices in tow and all would be right in the world.

The Everyday Challenges

That summer I was living in a house full of boys and sharing the master bedroom with Jill and our friend Danielle. I kept a mini fridge in our room to make sure I always had plenty of fresh produce on hand. A lifestyle consisting of daily green smoothies, fresh juice, and an abundance of steamed veggies and roasted vegetable soups called for a hell of a lot of produce. And when I say a hell of a lot, I mean enough to make a woman feeding a family of five look at me funny for the amount of produce in my grocery cart (that I bought biweekly, at least).

Living with so many people meant lots of different diets and lots of different aromas filling the house. When I ate meals from my regular plant-based diet, it didn't bother me to watch my roommates barbecue their chicken or sauté their fish, and so many of them were healthy eaters, we actually enjoyed a lot of the same foods. But those three days of juice cleansing were a very different story. One roommate of mine made quinoa and tilapia every night for dinner, and the overwhelmingly satisfying smell of his meal made me question what on earth I was doing drinking only juice for three days straight.

The crispy, flaky, lemony fish looked so dense and satiating I hardly knew what to do with myself. I must have mentioned how hungry I was a few times too many or a bit too vigorously because at one point Jill said, "Just eat if you're so hungry," to which I replied, "I'm on a cleanse." (It's really a surprise that no one killed me and/or kicked me out of our house during that time . . . seriously.)

While I was on the cleanse, I bounced back and forth between feeling on top of the world for having the willpower to drop 5 pounds (2.3 kg) in such a superhuman amount of time and feeling entirely and utterly fatigued and angry with myself for being so strict. I went out with my friends while they let loose, sipped on drinks, made snacks before bed, and went out for breakfast burritos the next morning, all the while shoving a straw into my green juice. People frequently made comments about how strict I was with myself, but my comeback to them and to myself was that they didn't have to deal with stomach problems like mine, so they couldn't possibly understand.

When it came time to eat solid food again after that first three-day cleanse, I was semi-panicked. Should I just keep juicing so I could maintain the weight loss and make sure the last three days of torture were super worth it? Or should I use this as an opportunity to wipe my slate clean and stick to just fruits and veggies to stay lean and remain totally in control? What ultimately ended up happening was a combination of the two. The morning after my cleanse ended, my sister Melissa, my brother-in-law Jeff, and my two nieces were picking me up to go to the airport to meet my parents and fly to Hawaii. Since they would be arriving around 6:30 a.m., I was in a state of catatonic dread about what this day would mean food-wise. Should I eat breakfast before they came so I would be satisfied until we were on the plane, where I would then have a snack? Or should I wait to eat breakfast until I'd been awake longer so I didn't end up accidentally eating more during the day because I'd eaten such an early breakfast?

To resolve my fears, I decided to pack a cooler of food three times the size of an average carry-on. I filled it to the brim, fretting that the place where we were staying wouldn't have organic produce or be able to accommodate my lifestyle. And let me tell you, grocery shopping for food items while you're withering away on a juice cleanse is not the most pleasant or productive experience in the world. For a predominantly raw and always gluten-free vegan, it's an hours-long process that only results in intense desire for all foods around you, coupled with putting something "indulgent" down and picking it back up a hundred times before deciding not to get it.

The morning we flew to Hawaii was the morning my family almost killed me. The four who picked me up struggled to act normal when they saw me barreling toward the car with a gigantic cooler. We all had to squeeze against each other the whole way to the airport for it to even fit. Jeff immediately started scheming with me about how to get my liquids through security. Isabella, my niece, who was nine at the time, was beside herself that I might get in trouble or be questioned by security for all my obscure food belongings. My sister just thought I was crazy.

When we got in line for security, Jeff started grilling me about what I was going to say to make sure I would be prepared when we got to the front of the line. When security started questioning me, Jeff respectfully explained that I had debilitating food allergies and needed to travel with an abundance of food for my vacation to be on the safe side. Security was unimpressed. They unzipped my bag to rifle through it, and it wasn't long before they found a serrated knife I had thrown in there to make sure I would be able to slice my avocado on the plane.

Shit. I had forgotten about that. My sister looked at me like I had lost my mind, and Jeff looked at me with an expression that read, "Ummm, you're on your own for this one." I tried to explain that I was delirious when I packed my bag that morning and wasn't even thinking about the fact that knives are illegal on airplanes. I urged security to take the knife in exchange for letting me have the rest of my food—food that had cost me way too much time and money to lose. In the end, they took a carton of almond milk and a few coconut yogurts—and the knife—but let me get by with most everything else.

up & down

"WHILE I WAS ON THE CLEANSE, I BOUNCED BACK AND FORTH BETWEEN FEELING ON TOP OF THE WORLD FOR HAVING SUCH WILLPOWER AND DROPPING 5 POUNDS (2.3 KG) IN SUCH A SUPERHUMAN AMOUNT OF TIME AND FEELING ENTIRELY AND UTTERLY FATIGUED AND ANGRY WITH MYSELF FOR BEING SO STRICT."

My entire family was waiting for me on the plane. "Please, dear God, tell me you didn't actually try to bring a knife on the plane," my mom said.

"I wasn't thinking!" I said, which was true, but I knew I had lost any and all validity at this point. All that really mattered to me, though, was I'd made it through the morning on only half a banana and one little scoop of almond butter. I was a bit nauseous, but hey, I was fresh off my three-day cleanse, which meant I was basically the equivalent of superwoman.

I remember each and every thing I ate from there on out on the trip, from some sliced pineapple on the plane to my carefully constructed green smoothies at the breakfast buffet. (I will add that I shed true tears of devastation when I found out that the protein powder they added to my smoothie was whey protein, also known as a milk, or non-vegan, product.)

I also remember that one night at dinner, my family ordered our hotel's signature "Ahi on a Rock" dish, where you have the option of searing the ahi yourself at your table or eating it raw. The big slab of tuna looked so juicy and delicious I could hardly handle it, but instead of trying it, I picked away at my vegetable brown rice—an indulgent dish for me no less—as I fielded my family's questions about why I ate less than a quarter of the meal and took the rest to go.

superwoman

"ALL THAT REALLY MATTERED TO ME, THOUGH, WAS I'D MADE IT THROUGH THE MORNING ON ONLY HALF A BANANA AND ONE LITTLE SCOOP OF ALMOND BUTTER. I WAS A BIT NAUSEOUS, BUT HEY, I WAS FRESH OFF MY THREE-DAY CLEANSE, WHICH MEANT I WAS BASICALLY THE EQUIVALENT OF SUPERWOMAN."

My propensity for taking food to go was a bit of a running joke in my circle of family and friends. I was always in a steady state of panic about not having enough vegan food on hand, so if I had something left over on my plate, which I always did because at the time I never finished my meals, you better believe I was going to take it home just to have it as an option. It also made me feel better about eating out; I could eat just a bit of my dish and save the rest for later. Mind you, it didn't matter to me if I actually did eat the rest, but having it on hand was strangely comforting, like having anxiety pills in your purse that you know you're not going to take or an emergency protein bar in your car that hasn't been touched for three years.

I spent the rest of the trip vacillating between feeling bloated from eating solid food postcleanse and feeling starved from the lack of nutrients and lack of variety in my diet. I hadn't reached full-fledged orthorexia yet, or at least I didn't realize it if I had, but I do remember eating a glorious slice of vegan cheesecake after dinner one night and feeling so sickly full from it that I both verbally and silently vowed to never eat dessert again.

On the way back home, I was supposed to fly back to LA with my sister, Jeff, and the girls while my parents flew to Northern California. But when we got to the airport, there was no record of a Jordan Younger on any flight. We argued and argued with the airline, and eventually they put me on a different flight, where I wasn't going to be with anyone in my family. I was twenty-two years old, so this wasn't really a big deal, but it was still annoying and jarring to change my flight plan. I said good-bye to them as they took off while I waited another three hours for my plane to arrive.

The Birth of *The Blonde Vegan*

Little did I know that those three hours would redefine my life as I knew it. As I sat curled up in my chair at the gate, surrounded by sun-kissed families with the end-of-vacation blues, I decided to create an Instagram account for my vegan food photos. I figured I had enough shots stored on my phone to create something interesting to look at for people who were reading up on health. Plus, I knew my friends were getting sick of seeing the rapidly increasing number of food photos on my personal account.

I chose the account name @theblondevegan, which I thought was playful yet straightforward, and embodied my personality just enough. (I also thought it might give people who knew me a little chuckle once they realized what I was doing.) And who knows, maybe, eventually, I would create a blog if there was enough interest.

I sat at the airport uploading photos, filtering them, and applying hashtags I saw other vegan food bloggers using on their photos: #whatveganseat, #plantbased, #plantstrong, #veganfoodporn, #veganfoodshare, #healthspo, and, of course, my new creation, #theblondevegan. I posted a screenshot of my new account on my existing personal Instagram. I wrote a caption telling my friends to follow if they were interested in seeing what I was up to in the vegan world.

By the time I landed in LA, I had about eighty followers and a few "Congrats!" and "This rocks!" comments sprinkled throughout from some extra-supportive friends. I even had a few followers who I didn't know, which I guessed was because of the hashtags. So I added a few more photos. And the next day I woke up with a small handful of new followers, both people I knew and people I didn't know.

I felt weirdly excited about this new project, and with two months to go before moving to New York and beginning graduate school, I had some time to dedicate to it. People in my life started to refer to me, somewhat jokingly but kind of seriously because it fit so well, as "TBV," and I thought it had a nice ring to it. It seemed like people were into it—and I certainly was—so why not keep it up?

Growing the account turned into a massive project. I looked at it through the creative lens with which I approached most things, and I saw what it took to grow my following each day. People liked colorful photos, but they also liked engagement. No one wants to support someone who isn't grateful for their following, so I made it a huge point to respond to each and every question and comment that came my way. At first it was easy to do, and it was extremely flattering. I couldn't believe people were so interested in my healthy-food ventures.

Every time I went out to eat, I ordered a colorful vegan dish and styled it on the table, moving the silverware and the water glasses out of the way or leaving them in if they were aesthetically pleasing enough. I also spent tons of hours in my parents' kitchen that summer, concocting all sorts of colorful layered oatmeal recipes and photographing bowls of overflowing berry and kale salads.

After a few weeks, I had my routine down to a science. I woke up, made some sort of plant-based dish that was different from the last, styled it, photographed it, and then went outside to post it where I had the best cell reception. Then I would hashtag the photo like crazy and start going to other people's photos to "like" and comment on them to bring people back to my new photo. I did the same thing with lunch and the same with dinner. The creative element excited me in a way I had never experienced. I knew what it was like to be passionate about health, writing and connecting with people, but never before had I been able to combine all those things and put my own artistic spin on it.

In a way, growing the Instagram account became an obsession as well, but aside from the food aspect, it wasn't an unhealthy obsession. It gave me something to focus on when I had the potential to be in a very difficult, transformative place. I had just graduated and was about to move across the country. Now, instead of panicking about what was to come, I could spend my time homing in on something I loved and developing a miniature brand for myself.

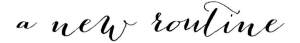

a new routine

"AFTER A FEW WEEKS, I HAD MY ROUTINE DOWN TO A SCIENCE. I WOKE UP, MADE SOME SORT OF PLANT-BASED DISH THAT WAS DIFFERENT FROM THE LAST, STYLED IT, PHOTOGRAPHED IT, AND THEN WENT OUTSIDE TO POST IT WHERE I HAD THE BEST CELL RECEPTION."

Once I saw that there was interest, I made up my mind that a blog had to happen. Instagram captions were not the best space to write an entire recipe, and with a blog, I could also write about my thoughts on health, fitness, yoga, nutrition, and anything else I felt like writing about. I had a built-in audience that seemed to be growing rapidly, and I knew I had to take advantage of the situation while it lasted. I had no idea if I would be able to keep it up with this much time and energy once grad school started, so I wanted to enjoy it while I still could.

I didn't know where to begin or have the slightest clue about how to use a blog platform. On Facebook, I asked if anyone I knew would be willing to help me create a website, and I heard right back from a friend of mine who I went to school with, Morgan Oliver-Allen. He said he had some experience with website design and would be happy to help me get started. We tossed around some ideas, and next thing I knew, he was working on logos.

The first time I saw the words *The Blonde Vegan* in logo form, I just about died. I couldn't believe my tiny little airport idea was turning into something more and more tangible by the day. We tossed around ideas for the "About" section, and I started sending him recipes and initial blog posts to put on the site so it would have some content once we launched it.

The first post was titled "*If you're reading this . . .* ," and when I sent it to Morgan, he laughed and told me how crazy long it was. I said I didn't care and that all my posts were probably going to be longer than other bloggers' because when I write, I write a *lot*. I knew people didn't have to

Tangible

"THE FIRST TIME I SAW THE WORDS *THE BLONDE VEGAN* IN LOGO FORM, I JUST ABOUT DIED. I COULDN'T BELIEVE MY TINY LITTLE AIRPORT IDEA WAS TURNING INTO SOMETHING MORE AND MORE TANGIBLE BY THE DAY."

Blog Excerpt

"I'm not asking you to agree with everything I say, and I'm certainly not asking you to go vegan if you don't have an interest in doing so, but I'm asking you to read this blog to gain a little insight into the life of a typical vegan gal. I am getting my MFA in creative writing, so I am a pretty decent writer too, I promise—I'm not going to be one of those bloggers that's like, "OK so like today I went to the mall and then I got my nails done and then my friends and I had a pool party." I want to write real stuff that inspires people and makes people think. And if I can ignite even the smallest spark inside you to do something you're passionate about, or if I can just make you smile or laugh, then this will all be worthwhile. Y'ALL READY? Because I am. This is going to be fun. Stay tuned for recipes and a whole lotta blog updates . . . I have been waiting to start a blog I have been passionate about for a LONG time. And if you've read this far, then I already love you."

read the whole thing if they didn't want to, but writing out my thoughts for other people to see felt so cathartic, I couldn't help but spill my guts. At that point, I didn't know if anyone would read it other than Morgan and my mom! But the act of doing it was what I enjoyed, and come fall, I'd have grad school to focus on anyway.

The day the blog launched was one of the most exciting days of my life. I had been telling my Instagram followers about it for weeks, and I knew that if even a couple of them clicked over to read it, I would be thrilled. The Instagram posting was fun, but it also felt kind of impersonal at times because no one knew what I looked like, how I talked, or that much about me or my personal life. I thought it would be cool to connect with my followers in a new way and offer them a bit of detail into who I was. The connection was such an important part to me.

Morgan made a beautiful site and basically brought my blog vision to life. So the morning I picked up and flew to New York to start the next chapter of my life, we launched the blog. I crafted a long and emotional Instagram post to debut it and anxiously awaited my followers' feedback. I didn't even know how to check the homepage of my hosting site, so Morgan reported back to me with the info. After the site had been up for an hour, he told me it had one thousand views, and he assured me that was a *lot* for the first hour of a blog's life.

"Jo, you might be able to do this for a living," he told me.

I was stunned. Only in my dreams would I be able to do such a thing! I told him I hoped he was right, but I knew there was a lot of work to do to get it to that point. I also knew I wouldn't always have the extra time on my hands to work on it like I did that first summer, but I still took it as a huge compliment and made a mental note that maybe, just maybe, I could make it happen one day.

Also, developing the blog had been incredibly good for my psyche. Even though all my photos were of plant-based food, my main focus was on styling the food and sharing the photos. Interacting with my readers, working on growing the site, and figuring out the most effective ways to reach people all became huge focuses in my life. Instead of someone who was just interested in health, nutrition, and fitness, I was now building a platform where I could share my knowledge.

It helped me to get out of my head and allowed me to view my lifestyle in a more global sense instead of in a self-obsessed or self-motivated way. I loved it, and I hoped I could continue to keep my focus on the entrepreneurial side of the blog once I got to New York.

5

MAKING NYC MY HOME
(A.K.A. NYC WHOLE FOODS TOUR)

After a summer spent developing *The Blonde Vegan*, it was time to jump into my MFA program. But instead of hopping from coffee shop to coffee shop and working on my novel, discussing literature, and getting to know my classmates, I spent most of my time brainstorming about TBV. Naturally, TBV was centered on plant-based food, so that took up a lot of space in my mind as well. And I wasn't the only one at The New School with a blog. Everyone there was passionate about writing, so most of them had blogs of their own, but from what I could gather, no one was quite as into it as I was. Plus, they definitely weren't into health blogging—I was the odd one out on that front.

My blog was still a baby, and even though I had encouragement from Morgan and a few other people about its potential for success, blogging as a career still wasn't really on my radar. I kept creating recipes, snapping photos, posting them to Instagram, and sending massively long blog entries for Morgan to post. Yes, it took several months for me to post on my own and even longer for a regular blogging schedule to develop. (I thought posting five-ish recipes at once was normal and didn't understand why each of those five never got as much traffic as when I posted one alone. Thanks to Morgan for telling me that's why, to this day, zero people have commented on my Quinoa Mac 'n' Cheese recipe!)

Even though blogging was becoming a huge part of my life, I was wide open to seeing what New York had to offer. I spent the first few weeks getting accustomed to my neighborhood and relishing the beauty of spending time *alone* for what felt like the first time in four years. I had a whole lot of time to spend with the few people I did know at that point, to get to know the vegan restaurants and juice/smoothie bars in the area, to start forming relationships with organic restaurant owners to interview on the blog, and to, of course, tour every nook and cranny of every Whole Foods Market in Manhattan.

I kept assuring my parents that once school officially started and the workload got heavier, the blog and my obsessive recipe developing and food photographing would take a backseat. But once school started and I saw everyone else around me working on their fiction full-time, my elaborate visions about sitting at charming cafés in the West Village and pouring my soul into my fictional characters' lives turned into me writing for twenty minutes at a time and then rushing home to create recipes and email with my readers.

That's when my obsession with the food aspect of my healthy lifestyle reemerged. I would be sitting in class but daydreaming about every possible pumpkin, oat, and almond butter combination to make a killer seasonal crumble and visualizing the layout I would create on my window ledge, the place with the best lighting in my apartment, to photograph it. Or I would be out at a bar with my friends after class sipping on a vodka soda but thinking neurotically about how early I would have to wake up to get to the gym before writing the next day, and how small a breakfast I would have to eat to feel light despite the alcohol.

obsession

"THAT'S WHEN MY OBSESSION WITH THE FOOD ASPECT
OF MY HEALTHY LIFESTYLE REEMERGED."

Finding a Vegan Voice

One of the greatest things about living in New York was living with my closest and oldest friend, Katie. We had talked about moving to NYC together after college for as many years as both of us could remember, but the fact that we made the dream a reality was still a shock to us both. Neither of us had ever lived away from California for a definitive period of time, but we were both ready for an adventure. If Katie hadn't been there during my year in New York, it would have been vastly different and not nearly as much fun. She knew me pretty much as well as I knew myself, and on many occasions she called me out for my increasingly weird eating habits. I had to be pretty sneaky if I was going to hide my health-driven idiosyncrasies from her.

When Katie introduced me to her coworkers at Tiffany's after we'd lived in New York for a few months, she described me as a food blogger rather than an MFA student. When I met new people in the city, I found myself rambling on and on about my "day job" as a health blogger versus my very serious ambitions of being a writer in the traditional sense of the word. More and more people I grew up with started associating me with my blog, and it got to the point where many people thought I'd moved to New York to pursue my blog and didn't even realize I was also in grad school.

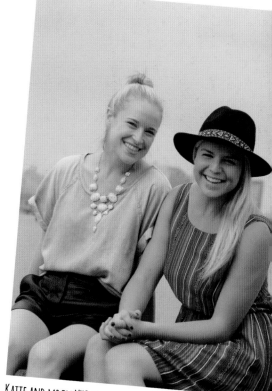

KATIE AND ME IN NYC AFTER LIVING THERE FOR A COUPLE OF WEEKS

It made sense to me that the blog was becoming such a focus in my life. It was *there*, and it was concrete. The fiction I was working on was so introspective, and I only got to share it with my classmates about twice a semester. In the blog world, I could write about my innermost fears, anxieties, desires, passions, and ideas, and I could put it all out into the world for immediate feedback. With Katie at work all day and most of my friends and family across the country, my blog readers kept me company. They were my coworkers and my confidants. If I didn't have a post to engage them with that day, I felt a little empty.

When I came across challenges like having a falling out with my professor or getting my heart broken, both of which happened exactly once in those early months in New York, it was the blog that I turned to. I wrote about my experiences and expressed every last detail of what I was feeling, whether through actual words or through what I created in the kitchen. My content creation depended on plant-based food, so my diet was hugely important.

I saw early on in my blogging career that writing about a specialty kind of food with a very niche audience was the key to rapidly growing success. I took healthy treats we all know and love like chocolate peanut butter cups and banana cream pie and made them healthy. I didn't make them "healthy" like a lot of the whole-wheat flour, applesauce instead of oil, brown sugar instead of white sugar recipes we've all seen cropping up over the years; I made them *healthy* as in every ingredient is bursting with nutrients that will fuel you and energize you instead of bog you down.

experiences

"I WROTE ABOUT MY EXPERIENCES AND EXPRESSED EVERY LAST DETAIL OF WHAT I WAS FEELING, WHETHER THROUGH ACTUAL WORDS OR THROUGH WHAT I CREATED IN THE KITCHEN."

I was enamored with making health more accessible to my readers and to people who didn't have access to it the same way I did. I had found this healthy way of living that changed my body and my quality of life, and I had somewhat accidentally stumbled upon this cyber outlet where I could share that passion with other people who wanted the same thing. Late nights responding to emails from readers replaced the late nights I imagined I would spend on creative bursts with the novel, and Friday nights on the couch writing my cleanse programs substituted for the barhopping I already found so repetitive and exhausting.

Soon enough I was getting emails from brands about sending me free product in exchange for blog posts. Score! I remember calling my mom to tell her about a partnership with Vega One, a protein powder company I had loved for a long time, with the excitement someone might have about winning the lottery. And at that point, I wasn't even getting paid for partnerships; I was just so thrilled that brands like Vega even knew my blog existed.

After creating content for that product post, which I learned to refer to as an "in-kind" partnership, I started getting opportunities to do more and more. Soon my tiny NYC kitchen was overflowing with free food. There were cold-pressed juices, natural energy bars, premade salads from local organic delivery services, endless jars of almond butter, and all sorts of superfood powders and vegan treats. In many cases, the foods sent to me were foods I would never dream of buying on my own. Some of the bars had cane sugar in them (gasp!), and the almond butters were often mixed with maple syrup, coconut sugar, and sometimes even chocolate chips.

Plus, the juices and smoothies had more fruit in them than I put in the smoothies I made in my own Vitamix, but I felt obligated to fully try everything before posting about it and endorsing it on the blog. It wasn't long before my regimented routine of a green smoothie for breakfast, a kale salad with berries for lunch, and roasted veggies with a grain for dinner was tipped out of whack by all these new goodies. To make up for the fullness I felt from trying everything, I started skipping meals every so often. A dinner here, a lunch there, a light green juice instead of a hearty veggie plate. It seemed innocent enough, and it was helping me maintain my low weight, so I didn't see a problem with it at first.

Maintaining Internal Balance

It felt strangely easy to eat less than my body wanted. In a way it was a response to the stress of maintaining my new lifestyle. I loved how new and exciting everything was, but it was also quite a departure from the life I was used to in California. I was used to being in college, living with my six best friends, and seeing my parents about twice a month. Now I was in a totally new environment and starting to grow a brand I was extremely passionate about. Not to mention the fact that I was experiencing a budding passion for food that was starting to verge on obsession. Reacting to all the newness by maintaining a stricter and stricter diet regimen seemed like a great stress outlet. It made me feel in control.

The physical aspect was also important to me. Eating plant-based, I felt like I had finally discovered the healthiest version of myself. Tiny, fit, strong Jordan reflected the Jordan who was passionate about health above all else. My body, in *my* mind, represented a health and fitness blogger who people could *trust* for nutrition and exercise advice. I started viewing all the free food crowding my kitchen space as somewhat dangerous to my diet and a little unwelcome.

I bounced back and forth between being really strict with my food intake and allowing myself to "live a little." Katie kept a close eye on me and tried to get me to make more of the veggie stir-fry dishes I loved instead of skipping them in favor of a juice. And whenever I ate the appropriate amounts my body craved, I gained a few pounds (1 to 2 kg) and my stomach problems started to come back. I didn't understand why the veggies weren't soothing my stomach like they once had. Every morning I told myself if I just started the day with a small green smoothie, then I would be able to get back on track.

It's startling for me now to think that I felt self-conscious about my weight at that time. I had gained a few pounds (1 to 2 kg) since the very beginning of my vegan days, but I was still thinner than my body is meant to be. My gaunt face and tiny frame speak for themselves when I look at photos from my first few months in New York. I was beginning to lose the natural coloring in my face from so many months on purely fruits and veggies, and I was exercising like a maniac. I was the opposite of big, but that's exactly how I felt.

The three pounds (1.4 kg) between me and my "goal weight," also known as the weight I had been earlier that year when I first went vegan, felt like the difference between petite and huge. I knew it was irrational, but when I looked in the mirror or put on my jeans, those few extra pounds (1 to 2 kg) were all I could see or feel. Avoiding the food that was sent to me to review by taking a bite instead of eating a whole bar or by taking a sip of a smoothie rather than finishing it, felt like a victory, and oh my, I was determined to be victorious.

I looked incessantly through photos of myself from college to remind myself that though I had a few pounds (1 to 2 kg) I wanted to lose, I was significantly smaller than I had been when I was a free-for-all-binge-drinking-3 a.m.-queso-dip-inhaling college student. And when I drank a green smoothie full to the brim and felt like an overly full failure, I reminded myself that a sixteen-ounce (475 ml) green smoothie was nothing in comparison to the sandwiches on focaccia or the spinach and cheese ravioli that used to characterize a typical lunch or dinner for me.

I was in a constant internal battle between feeling good about my lifestyle and panicking about gaining weight or eating something that might make my stomach problems return. If I felt even the slightest hint of indigestion coming on, I deemed whatever food I had just eaten untouchable and promised myself never to go anywhere near it again.

victory

"AVOIDING THE FOOD THAT WAS SENT TO ME TO REVIEW BY TAKING A BITE INSTEAD OF EATING A WHOLE BAR OR BY TAKING A SIP OF A SMOOTHIE RATHER THAN FINISHING IT FELT LIKE A VICTORY, AND OH MY, I WAS DETERMINED TO BE VICTORIOUS."

I was often praised for the willpower and self-control I exhibited to maintain my strict diet, and I absolutely loved it. When my parents came to visit for my twenty-third birthday, they took me and a group of friends out to dinner at Buddakan in Chelsea, my longtime favorite restaurant. Buddakan has an incredible menu of pan-Asian cuisine, delicious cocktails, and tons of different dishes suitable for vegans and non-vegans alike. My parents ordered a tasting menu for the table that included enough food to feed twenty-five people (we were a party of seven), but of course, I had to order all my own vegan food on top of it because my preferences didn't exactly fall in line with everyone else's.

High on the celebratory vibes, I ate veggies and tofu slathered in rich sauces and drank mint-muddled cocktails to my heart's content. When the desserts came, of which there were about ten thanks to the tasting menu, I was cajoled into taking a bite of a NON-VEGAN chocolate cake. And when I say a bite, I mean a nibble so small a mouse would hardly be able to scavenge it off the ground.

However, that bite, along with the generous helpings of everything else I had eaten that night (vegan, yes; healthy, eh) left me feeling so guilty I was sure I had broken some kind of healthy-living, plant-based vegan rule. I vividly remember sitting in my faux leather dress, my thinning blonde locks draped over my shoulders, trying hard to smile and join in the fun but thinking ever so clearly: "I am a fat cow because of everything I just ate."

pride

"MY LIPS WERE BLUE, AND I HAD SOMEHOW CONVINCED MYSELF THAT THE INDIGO COLOR THEY HAD TAKEN ON WAS A SIGN OF STRENGTH RATHER THAN A DISPLAY OF PURE NUTRIENT DEFICIENCY. EVEN THOUGH I WAS SO UNCOMFORTABLY COLD MY BONES HURT, I HAD PRIDE."

The next morning I woke up so strongly resolved to go back to my extremely healthy ways, I basically wanted my parents up and out and on a plane back to California if it meant I could restrict my food intake and hit the gym for a few hours. We went to brunch the next morning and I ordered oatmeal, another meal that was indulgent in my mind. Grains were a total treat because I hardly ever allowed myself to eat them. My parents and Katie all munched away on eggs Benedict and huevos rancheros, enjoying their food as usual and clearly not obsessing at all, and meanwhile, I spooned away at my oatmeal, feeling guiltier and guiltier with every bite.

"Don't you miss eggs?" Katie asked me while we were all eating. Everyone looked at me. They all knew what an egg fan I had been pre-veganism. "NO," I said, my go-to response. "I like the way I eat. That's why I eat this way. I really don't miss anything."

Goodness, was I pleasant to be around. And after the oatmeal "incident," I went back into my fruit, veggie, and occasional grain dietary mode like there was no tomorrow. If I ever found it difficult to maintain, I channeled the pain I felt from anything challenging going on in my life or just tried to put myself in a headspace where restricting made sense. Restricting meant being empty, and empty meant feeling good. Feeling good meant being tiny, and tiny meant having the utmost confidence. It. Made. Sense.

My birthday is in October, which means the very beginnings of chilliness were starting to sweep their way into the East Coast. I was a protein-deficient, frozen block of ice. My fingers had zero feeling in them at all times. My lips were blue, and I had somehow convinced myself that the indigo color they had taken on was a sign of strength rather than a display of pure nutrient deficiency. Even though I was so uncomfortably cold my bones hurt, I had pride.

My parents flew back to California, and I spent the next few months falling deeper and deeper into my restriction, baking seasonal desserts for the blog that I threw away after photographing because having them around made me anxious and continuing to disregard my schoolwork in favor of blogging. I still maintained a pretty unassuming front on the outside, but my food obsessions were slowly taking hold of my mind and becoming harder and harder to ignore.

6

THE HOLIDAYS: AN ORTHOREXIC'S WORST NIGHTMARE

Come holiday time, I was beginning to figure out how to monetize the blog. And believe you me, doing so was necessary because the amount of time I spent working on it far surpassed a socially acceptable quantity to not be getting paid. I was doing product review posts here and there, but product reviews seemed so *obvious* and also boring to read compared to the yummy recipe posts and juicy lifestyle tidbits I liked to write.

So instead of going to town on the sponsored posts for the sake of making money, I decided to create a plant-based cleanse program to sell through the blog. It would cover all the basics: how to cleanse, why to cleanse, when to cleanse, where to buy organic produce, and, of course, I would then be able put on paper and share with others one more thing I was insanely obsessed with—cleansing. The program consisted of five recipes per day: one smoothie, two juices, and two solid food meals. The meals were made purely from fruits, veggies, and nuts and were mainly salads, soups, and roasted vegetable dishes. (Does the cleanse program sound familiar? It was based on the five-day plant-based cleanse I did with my mom one year prior—the cleanse that turned me on to plant-based veganism in the first place.)

I set to work writing the twenty-five recipes, photographing them, and including blog-style summaries and nutritional information for each one. The cleanse was my first professional engagement with an outside source, other than my TBV web designer, and after one major trial-and error-experience, I ended up working with a close friend from high school to do the graphic design. She brought my vision to life beautifully, and I was so excited to start selling it, I didn't know how I could possibly wait until the week before the new year to release it.

I was solidly convinced that whoever tried the cleanse would become hooked on living a plant-based lifestyle. I thought that if people would just give veganism a try, there's no way they couldn't fall as head over heels in love with it as I had. How could anyone resist feeling so freaking light and in control of what they were putting into their bodies?

Another major excitement about the cleanse was that I would finally have a group of people to go through the cleansing process with me. I had done the five-day cleanse with my mom in the past and I had a few friends who were interested in trying one-day juice cleanses with me, but this would be different. It would be a group of people from all over the world offering sup-port, motivation, and advice. I couldn't wait to get started with them and for all of us to inspire each other. I also couldn't wait to feed off their motivation and to cleanse my heart out. I was desperately hoping that cleansing this time around would help me find my balance again.

Also, I was extremely happy to have a month-long break from school and to be back home with my family in Northern California for a few weeks. The holidays have always been my favorite time of year, and even though I was semi-panicked about navigating my first holiday season as a vegan, I was so happy to be out of the freezing cold for a while, it hardly mattered. I wasn't sure how I was going to find the motivation to go back to school and continue putting energy into it while my heart was so much more in line with the blog.

It was tough to blog when I was surrounded by people in my grad school program who looked down on blogging as if it had no real value. Some of the traditional poets and fiction writers in my workshop classes gave me attitude about how much time I spent blogging. I once did a project on blogging as an art form and was basically torn apart by some of my class-mates and even my professor. They didn't understand how it matched up to the literary efforts of writing in the traditional sense, and they mocked the top-read bloggers in my presentation by saying their writing meant nothing because it was superficial and little to no editing was involved.

Their criticism was hard to take and made me feel very out of place in the scheme of the program. I had some amazing friends in my classes who defended me when people questioned my blogging career, but at the end of the day, I knew what I was passionate about, and it wasn't grad school. The negative way the literary community in New York perceived blogging only drove me to blog more and continue developing the business side of my brand. I didn't feel like I needed to prove them wrong, but I needed to see for myself that what I was spending so much time working on was legitimate enough to be a lasting creative outlet. Blogging came so much more naturally to me at this stage of my life than working on my fiction did, so I hoped it had as much promise as it seemed to. I didn't want to ditch my fiction endeavors entirely, but I was definitely flirting with the idea of putting them on the back burner for a while.

Cleansing for Power

With my mind swimming in confusion about my next move with grad school, I was very eager to start the cleanse on the first of the year and exercise control over my life in that way. I knew seeing the number on the scale go down would feel like a direct correlation to my willpower and my dedication to a healthy lifestyle, and I couldn't wait to feel that feeling. I didn't love having my mental state tied in so intricately with my diet choices, but I didn't think it was something I could change. I had already devoted myself to living as healthy as possible, so it only seemed natural that I would want to be as "healthy" (a.k.a. clean and pure) as I could.

I tried to do other things I thought would make me feel happy and in control to see if I could help the healthy-food obsession fade. I dyed my hair dark at the roots (very dark), thinking that sort of drastic change might excite me the same way controlling my food intake did. It didn't have nearly the same effect. It was a big change, but without that empty feeling in my stomach to back it up, I didn't feel accomplished in the same way that a cleanse or restriction made me feel.

The week of Christmas, my sister brought me a box of vegan peanut butter cookies from her local farmer's market. She had been raving to me about them for months and couldn't wait for me to try them. I immediately panicked. I could see the brown sugar gleaming on them in the harsh kitchen light. The ingredients were minimal, but they still didn't fall under my fully plant-based mental requirements. Even having them in the house and knowing they were there for me filled my chest with anxiety.

My family nibbled on the cookies throughout the week, and I say "nibbled" because there were far more indulgent and delicious desserts in the house, and most of my family couldn't have cared less about those organic, local, vegan, almost-but-not-quite-sugar-free cookies on the countertop. They looked really good, they smelled amazing, and I have always been a sucker for anything involving peanut butter and chocolate chips. But something very strong in my mind held me back from trying them, and I knew I wasn't going to go anywhere near them. I also hoped no one was going to notice and ask me about it because I knew my rationale made no sense. It didn't even make sense to me. I didn't understand where my mental blockage was coming from, other than the intense fear of my stomach pain returning with a vengeance because of trying something new.

On Christmas Day, I decided to give myself a bit of a breakfast treat—it was a holiday, after all—and make a coconut yogurt parfait with granola while my family ate what we have every year for breakfast Christmas morning: my mom's scrambled eggs, sausage, and English muffins. I constructed the parfait carefully, mindful of enjoying the aromas and the textures because I knew that was supposed to make the overall experience of eating more satisfactory. I ate the whole thing, all the while feeling kind of sad and nostalgic that I couldn't join in on our breakfast tradition, and afterward I obsessed so much about the amount of food I ate, I ended up feeling extremely nauseous and bloated.

Naturally, everyone else felt great.

anxiety

"EVEN HAVING [THE COOKIES] IN THE HOUSE AND KNOWING THEY WERE FOR ME FILLED MY CHEST WITH ANXIETY."

I was not happy. I was trying to be the one prioritizing my health, and I was the only one feeling terrible and wanting to curl up in the fetal position on my bed. That little setback sent me into somewhat of a tailspin. It started with a few "I don't feel good" remarks to my mom whenever she would walk by, and then a "My stomach really hurts" to whoever would listen, and then "Okay, I'm officially worried" at the top of my lungs to the entire household. They were not amused, and the rant was also nothing new because they'd been hearing about my stomach problems my entire life.

But this time it felt different and even more wrong than what I was used to. There I was paying serious attention to every single bite that went into my mouth, and I was still suffering from the same stomach problems I so intensely believed veganism had cured. I spent the whole day in and out of tears and wailing about how unfair it was that I had to be so careful about what I ate when everyone else could just enjoy food and go on with their lives as normal. I became even more fixated on starting the plant-based cleanse come January 1, and hell, why not start even sooner? I thought that maybe by doing the same thing I had done when I began my vegan journey, I would be able to reap the benefits again.

People didn't even know what to do with me anymore. I was the strictest eater nearly anyone in my life had ever known, yet I hardly ever felt good. I know now that the extreme focus I was putting on my diet was making my stomach pain and anxiety ten times worse than it should have been, but I also know now that the vegan diet was no longer working for me and my body was doing everything in its power to tell me so. Instead of listening, I obsessed over starting the cleanse again. No matter how hard I tried to enjoy being home with my family and out of the harsh East Coast winter, beginning the cleanse was the *only* thing on my mind that holiday season.

strict

"PEOPLE DIDN'T EVEN KNOW WHAT TO DO WITH ME ANYMORE. I WAS THE STRICTEST EATER NEARLY ANYONE IN MY LIFE HAD EVER KNOWN, YET I HARDLY EVER FELT GOOD."

Something I can also see with clarity now is that writing the cleanse and then running an email thread throughout the week for all the cleanse participants was one of the catalysts that tipped me over the edge from food obsession into full-blown orthorexia. I already focused on health food in my mind and on the blog, and now hundreds upon hundreds of people wanted to discuss cleansing with me, talk about the fruit and veggie recipes, and hire me to create more.

Oh, and the amount of money I made selling the cleanse at $25 per person was the first time I had ever made a reasonable amount of money in my life. So not only was I encouraged by my readers to create more cleanses, but also by my family and pretty much anyone with half a brain when it comes to managing a business. From that month forward, I marketed the cleanse like a madwoman. I cleansed with my readers the first week of every month, and selling it became my main source of income.

My confidence in my willpower around food resurged during that first week of January. I'd had weeks to prepare for the restriction, and while I truly believed the cleanse was helping my readers get healthier and learn what it was like to live a processed-free, meat-free week, for me it was so much more. It was a rededication to my lifestyle, and it was the proof I needed that if I restricted just enough, my stomach problems would remain at bay.

For some reason, when I was on a "cleanse," it was much easier to stick to really small portions and to substitute juices and smoothies for meals. I think that's because my self-control was a total mental state at that time. There was not a whole lot of mind-body connection going on. If my body was giving me hunger cues, I was doing my best to ignore them. If my exhaustion indicated that I wasn't giving myself enough fuel and nourishment, I didn't believe it. I was on a mission to be totally *pure*, and I wasn't going to let any kind of doubt get in the way. Doubt did not exist in my mind. I was all in.

7

JUICE CLEANSING & THE RAW VEGAN LIFE

My new-year plant-based cleanse reaffirmed what I already knew: Juice cleansing made me feel on top of the world.

After my initial bouts with solid-food plant-based cleansing and a couple of three-day juice cleanses (remember my end-of-college cleanse pre–Hawaii trip?), I knew that putting myself on any sort of cleanse would make me feel good again even if I had been feeling super off-balance. I advocated juice cleanses for all the right reasons, warned people against using them as a quick fix to get healthy, and loudly proclaimed that they aren't *sustainable* methods of losing weight (*psh*, who does that?), but per usual, I wasn't exactly living by my own advice.

I will always remember stepping on the scale every thirty minutes during my first three-day juice cleanse and feeling somewhat herculean watching the number creep down lower and lower each day. "Hell yeah, gaining weight isn't even a *thing* when you're this healthy," I believed while giving myself a mental high five and anxiously awaiting the two-hour mark to chug down my next juice.

But even then, even when I was sipping on lemon cayenne water and dreaming of inhaling the tilapia and quinoa whose aromas filled my desperately starving nostrils, I hadn't let the juice cleanses take over my being. I did that initial three-day juice cleanse in June and didn't do another full-blown cleanse until the next fall. I've always been one to pay a pretty penny for good quality, nourishing organic products, but juice cleanses are pretty damn expensive for a barely employed postgrad, so they weren't exactly on my weekly radar, until . . .

That's right. Until I started getting them offered to me by the dozens. TBV was like a breeding ground for juice companies and juice bars to get free advertising, and hey, why would I not take advantage of every cleanse offered? Cleansing made me healthy! Cleansing made me thin! Cleansing made my very abnormal digestion run like clockwork! Cleansing made me feel like a freaking champion who didn't need solid food to succeed in life, and I was going to prove it to myself, and to anyone watching, again and again.

So there I was, this little blonde Californian transplant in the harshest winter New York City had seen since the sixties, and I was determined to live predominantly on liquids. Juicing filled me with a strange sense of ease because I didn't have to cook, and as a plant-based vegan blogger, cooking took up a fair amount of my time. Or at least that's why I thought juicing made me feel more relaxed.

Somewhere in the back of my mind, I knew it wasn't just the spare time on my hands that made me feel so much calmer while on a juice cleanse. It was the fact that I didn't have to think about food at *all*. The thoughts about food that were beginning to plague my mind every day could be put to rest while I was on a juice cleanse, and my headspace was then cleared up enough to think about everything else going on in my life. Grad school, relationships, the growing blog, my new NYC life, yoga, training for my half marathon, keeping in touch with my California people, you know . . . the things I should have been able to focus on all along.

And on top of that, the anxiety constantly bubbling up in my insides had nothing to cling to in my stomach when there was no food in it. With nothing to hold on to, it kind of had no choice but to disappear or at least save itself for a later date. I learned to associate that empty feeling with a sense of serenity I became addicted to. When I wasn't wasting so much energy on stressing out and focusing on my stomach turning into a jumbled mess, I had more energy to live my life.

The "cleansing high" felt ridiculously good in the beginning. I was able to take the newfound energy I wasn't using on worrying about food and channel it into things I loved. After my first cleanse when I still lived in LA, I remember running into my bedroom on a weird starvation energy high and talking on the phone with Katie, long before we moved to New York together, and assuring her I was "happier than I have EVER been!" and

"Who needs [ex-boyfriend] anyway?!" and "I am finally living my true passions! I'm so HAPPY!" while throwing myself into a shoulder stand on my bedroom floor. (Literally.)

Katie sounded alarmed—supportive, but alarmed. And for good reason. I was a slowly deteriorating train wreck. Little did she know that one year later we would be living in a 450 square-foot (42 square meter) glorified box together in the West Village and our refrigerator would be overflowing with twenty-five juices at a time to feed my cleansing addiction; nor did she know that if she accidentally ate one of the bananas I was saving for a smoothie, I would flip out in a way that made little to no sense. (Especially considering there were three juice bars on our block alone and three grocery stores within a 0.1-mile [0.2 km] radius.)

Cleansing became my number one vice that winter, as well as my absolute go-to whenever anything felt like it was going wrong. I went to lectures by leaders in the raw vegan world, and many of them drew on the same points and principles; When we eat food that is not good for us, it will decompose in our stomachs and we will feel sick. To feel good, we must eat an abundance of raw fruits and veggies, combine them well, and drink lots and lots of fresh organic cold-pressed juice. Eating too many nuts is not good for your digestion. Combining the wrong fruits and veggies is *not* good for your digestion. Cooked food, even veggies, has little to no nutrients. Eating too much/eating too little/eating too often/not eating often enough are not good for you, and you will not be able to reap the benefits of a raw vegan diet.

What were my thoughts? Oh, shit. I'd better drink a ton of green juice and avoid nuts and cooked food and anything that might possibly make my stomach feel painful or overly full or, God forbid, bloated. And when I was

energy high

"I REMEMBER RUNNING INTO MY BEDROOM ON A WEIRD STARVATION ENERGY HIGH AND TALKING ON THE PHONE WITH KATIE, LONG BEFORE WE MOVED TO NEW YORK TOGETHER, AND ASSURING HER I WAS 'HAPPIER THAN I HAVE EVER BEEN!'"

slaving away writing *The Blonde Vegan Cleanse*, writing my novel for grad school, taking on every partnership offered to me on TBV, drawing up plans for TBV Apparel, staying on top of the massive amount of email flooding into in my inbox every day, and responding to social media and blog comments, I knew juicing was the answer. If I could avoid eating food that might decompose in my stomach and distract me from my work, then I believed I was doing something right.

So I juiced. And I juiced and I juiced and I occasionally blended. Once in a while, I would gorge on a raw vegan dessert from one of the many raw food cafés in our neighborhood. I would then feel like a complete failure, and more than likely, I would throw it right back up. Yes, I made myself throw up. This wasn't something that became a habit, but I did it every so often when I felt like I had lost control. I was willing to do anything to feel lighter and more in touch with my willpower.

A New Role Model

I attended one lecture in particular that struck a chord within me and made me extra enchanted by juice cleanses. At this point, I had been vegan for about a year and a half, and the plant-induced euphoria that initially made me feel incredible had long worn off. I was constantly trying new things to get back to that state of calmness in my stomach and peace in my mind. I was sick of fretting so terribly about every single bite that went into my body, and I just wanted a break from the compulsiveness.

Then along came this lecture about raw veganism and juicing. A juice company in New York was holding the event, and the speaker was someone I looked up to in the raw vegan community. He was in his eighties, thin as a rail, quick as a whip, and very passionate about all things raw veganism.

I remember everything about the morning I listened to him speak, down to what I was wearing, what I was doing afterward, and my level of hunger before, during, and after the event. I arrived early and snagged a front-row center seat, but not before buying a green juice in the front of the store to sip on during the lecture—for breakfast, duh. I was decked out in my new cuffed camo jeans and a "Health is the New Black" tank top from the TBV Apparel clothing line I'd just launched. I thought it would be a good idea to wear the shirt to a lecture about *health* and wrongly assumed everyone in the room would run up to me dying to know where I'd gotten it.

In truth no one cared or even noticed what I was wearing because everyone in the room was strangely mesmerized by the words of this raw vegan man, including me. He was agile as ever for his age, and his wispy white hair was brushed to the side like a California surfer boy. He put on a PowerPoint presentation about how he changed his life decades before that by finding raw veganism, and he spoke about the power of uncooked, organic plant-based foods in the authoritative way a lawyer defends his case.

He spoke about the benefits of probiotics, living raw, and the importance of cold-pressed green juice. All that was interesting enough to me, but what I really took away from the lecture was the way he spoke about juice cleansing. He had cleansed for over *one hundred* days at a time, living purely on cold-pressed juice—no solid foods at all. He ran marathons while he cleansed, and he described waking up the morning of a marathon and eating nothing because his body was still running on the fuel of his raw vegan meals from the days leading up to the race. Then he would have people meet him along the way and bring him dates (the dried fruit) and bananas.

I was *astounded*. I mean, call me naïve, but I was a plant-based vegan girl with fears of non-vegan foods, controlling her life through plants and teetering on the edge of developing a full-blown psychiatric problem. If someone was going to tell me they had found the magic ticket to health and it did *not* involve eating something I was afraid of, then I was all in. Plus, I was training for a half marathon, so by the end of his talk, I was already fantasizing about my pre-race starvation method and the great abundance of energy it would give me.

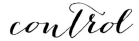

control

"I WAS *ASTOUNDED*. I MEAN, CALL ME NAÏVE, BUT I WAS A PLANT-BASED VEGAN GIRL WITH FEARS OF NON-VEGAN FOODS, CONTROLLING HER LIFE THROUGH PLANTS AND TEETERING ON THE EDGE OF DEVELOPING A FULL-BLOWN PSYCHIATRIC PROBLEM."

The main takeaway of the lecture for me was that juice cleanses are not effective unless you cleanse for weeks on end. Three-day cleanses made popular by health-conscious celebs and the mainstream media weren't going to cut it as far as our organs were concerned. And even though I'm a smart girl and I *knew* this lecture was being sponsored by a juice company that wanted nothing more than to sell extended juice cleanses to people in the audience, I soaked in his words as if he were my new raw vegan prophet.

So what did I do? I marched right up to the owner of the juice bar and the rest of his team, whom I worked with frequently on the blog, and I told them to count me in for an extended juice cleanse. It was a Saturday morning, and I wanted to start on Monday. I told them I would promote their company three times per day on my social media. I was basically willing to do anything if it meant I could start right away. The sooner the better . . . there was no way I was going back to eating cooked solid food if I had the option to cleanse—not after this lecture.

They agreed that the cleanse was a great idea, and we decided I would commit to thirty days, and of course, blog about it the whole time. For a second, I wondered how I was going to keep the interest of my blog readers and social media followers when the only food photos I would be able to post would be the same juices over and over again, but my concern was far outweighed by the excitement of this new challenge. I was beyond ready to test my superhuman willpower abilities and be well on the way to matching the health and exuberance of this wonderful eighty-five-year-old man I had just spent two hours listening to.

(Excuse me while I make a mental note to never, ever make a huge lifestyle decision based on someone else's body and their needs again. Comparing myself to other people in the health community and the multitude of diets they follow and swear by is one of the prime reasons I developed orthorexia.)

Regardless, I was stoked to try this majorly extended cleanse. In my mind, I would finally be joining the ranks of the raw vegan elite I so admired. Images of a leaner, fitter, tanner (don't ask) me floated through my mind and served as the motivation I needed to embark on this major lifestyle change—or starvation diet, whatever you prefer to call it.

I got home that day and eagerly—*too* eagerly—told Katie about my long-term cleansing plans. Can you guess what she did? She looked at me like I was insane, and not only that, she was kind of upset. She knew my mom and my sister were coming to visit in a few weeks, and then our other best friend, Danielle, was coming to stay with us. "You *can't* be on a cleanse when Danielle gets here," she said, insinuating that we wouldn't be able to do anything fun if I was cleansing.

I assured her that I wouldn't let my cleanse get in the way of anything we did with Danielle, and that regardless, I probably wasn't going to drink or be very adventurous in my food choices to begin with. I argued that really it would make things easier on everyone if I could just cart my juices around while Danielle visited. That way we could eat anywhere and do anything without having to worry about finding restaurants that accommodated my various limitations.

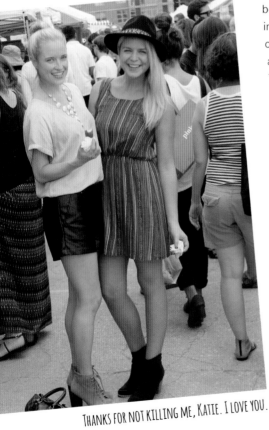

THANKS FOR NOT KILLING ME, KATIE. I LOVE YOU.

Katie more or less dropped it from there because she knew there was no reasoning with me. Once I was caught up in my one-track, health-addicted mindset, nothing anyone said would change my mind. That's a product of both who I am as a person and the strong hold my eating disorder was beginning to have on me. Once I made a decision, especially if it involved food or the promise of food restriction, there was absolutely no swaying me otherwise.

Plus, to add to the rocky relationship I was developing with solid food in general, at the time, I was seeing a plant-based nutritionist who advocated a three-meal-per-day plan where I was not supposed to snack in between meals or have anything sweet at all—including dried fruit. He drastically cut down the servings of fruit I could have from my previous unlimited amount (it was one of the only things I ate!) to three servings per day. According to his plan, I was supposed to steam my veggies instead of roasting them, and I was to have a large—in his words, "so large it would make people stare"—salad of purely leafy greens with both lunch and dinner.

I was seeing him in an attempt to get back on track with my stomach problems. I was still eating a diet of fruits, veggies, nuts, and the occasional grain and legume, but I was feeling nauseous a lot and more bloated than ever. I figured it must have had something to do with the food-combining rules I read so much about, and potentially a food sensitivity or two I wasn't aware of. A part of me was open to the idea of reintroducing eggs and fish into my diet every so often if it would help, and I kind of hoped the nutritionist would give me the green light to do that.

Instead, he told me I didn't need animal protein to thrive and be healthy. He suggested cleaning up my routine and regulating my meals instead. Another thing he told me was that it sounded like I have a nervous stomach (and I do), and that to combat it I should not eat anything when my stomach feels anxious. Well, shit. That meant I should rarely be eating at all because most of the time my stomach was an anxious mess.

He described how food does not digest properly when you eat on a nervous stomach and how it will then start decomposing, fermenting, and causing discomfort instead of giving you the nutrients you need. What?! The thought of food rotting in my sensitive tummy terrified me, so I resolved to eat as little as possible and replace meals with juices as often as I could—cleanse or no cleanse.

mindset

"ONCE I WAS CAUGHT UP IN MY ONE-TRACK, HEALTH-ADDICTED MINDSET, NOTHING ANYONE SAID WOULD CHANGE MY MIND. THAT'S A PRODUCT OF BOTH WHO I AM AS A PERSON AND THE STRONGHOLD MY EATING DISORDER WAS BEGINNING TO HAVE ON ME."

Family Heartbreak

And as if I were not already anxious enough, another part of my world that I had no control over seemed to be falling apart. Someone my dad worked with had involved him in a twisted business scheme that was not only devastating on a professional level, but was a *huge* betrayal of trust. It was the type of act that up until then I had only read about or seen in wild criminal documentaries that I had long been obsessed with watching. And now it was happening to us.

When I was given the news, I felt like all the wind had been knocked out of my body. Not my dad, I thought. There was no way someone could possibly do that to him. My dad is brilliant, and he is the kindest, most humble, and hardworking man I have ever known. To think that someone could turn on him in such an evil and shocking way rushed me, and it made me skeptical about anything and anyone I trusted in general.

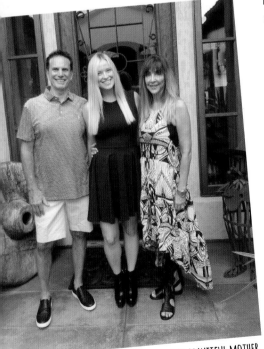

MY TWO ROCKS: MY INCREDIBLE FATHER AND BEAUTIFUL MOTHER. THANK YOU FOR ABSOLUTELY EVERYTHING.

From there on out, I felt perpetually sick. All I could think about was my dad, what this might mean for him, how sick and heartbroken he was, and how terrible some people in this world can be. A shift took place inside me that day. My trusting nature now had a huge dent in it, and it served as a reminder that life as I knew it could be stripped away in an instant.

So I did what I do best: I controlled through food. I stayed up late into the night researching raw veganism, the 80/10/10 diet, and "raw till 4," and writing meal plans for myself to follow. And then I started my thirty-day juice cleanse and wholeheartedly believed it would be the answer to my problems. If I wasn't eating, food would have no way to make me feel so sick all the time. And if there was nothing to digest, the perpetual swirls of anxiety might calm down and allow me to breathe a little easier.

I also needed a way to express my anger and frustration about the situation, and by this point I was so used to using my physical body as an expression of how I was feeling. When I was sad, I lost a few pounds (1 to 2 kg). When I was happy, I was lean and strong. And when I was depressed for more unexplainable reasons, I tried as hard as I could to maintain willpower so I could express my inner strength when my outer strength no longer existed.

But it was also through this extreme control that I started to see something I knew deep in my rational heart all along. Controlling my life through food wasn't going to make me feel any better when the problems I faced were real and concrete. My undying willpower to restrict was something I could latch on to when things got hard, but it wasn't reality. It was all in my head, and the moment my mind was taken over by hunger or stress or any tangible, present-moment feeling, restriction was no longer sustainable. It put so much pressure on me, I felt like I could break at the mere thought of continuing to go through the motions.

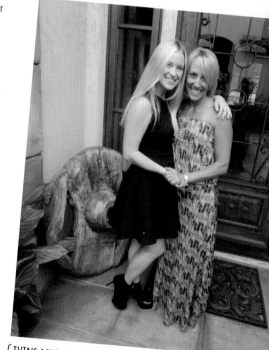

I knew I needed to make a change, or even several changes. I just didn't know yet what those changes were going to look like.

GIVING MY SISTER MELISSA A LITTLE SQUEEZE. LOVE YOU.

8

DOWN THE RABBIT HOLE

The issue of weight comes up *a lot* when I tell people my story. Most people think traditional eating disorders are based on fixation with weight loss. I will definitely acknowledge that the weight loss aspect of my strict plant-based diet was addictive. I loved that my thin, fit frame exuded the boundless clean-eating regimen I followed and the downright *emptiness* I felt on the inside. I was so attuned to my body's reaction to anything I ate or drank, I had programmed myself to panic whenever I felt "too full." Being full meant feeling guilty, and feeling guilty meant being washed over with a deep regret for what I had just eaten.

But controlling my food intake was about so much more than the weight itself. My low weight represented my control, my willpower, and my rigidity. It also gave me something to focus on when things in my personal and family life felt like too much to handle. I could only be strict with myself for so long before I started craving the acknowledgment that I did, in fact, look as thin and empty as I felt. If ever weeks or months went by without someone mentioning my efforts, I felt a little discouraged. I constantly flipped through old photos of myself, especially from my college study-abroad days, to show myself that I had come so far, and even if I was feeling guilty after eating a few too many handfuls of granola or juicy dates with almond butter, I was noticeably tinier, damn it.

Juice cleansing seemed like the most effective way to control my weight. I could drop seven to ten pounds (3.2 to 4.5 kg) in one week while I was on a cleanse, and even though I was the first to warn people against the unsustainability of quick-fix weight loss, it didn't stop me from getting hooked on doing it when I needed something to focus on that felt manageable and within reach. Controlling my life through food, at times, seemed frighteningly easy. My thirty-day juice cleanse started out innocently enough. I was desperate to cure my stomach problems and avoid solid food. I was fresh off my inspiration from the raw vegan lecture *and* newly aware that food could decompose in my nervous stomach; there was not a chance I was going to risk overeating solid food. Since the cleanse was going to be so long, I decided to "allow" myself one smoothie per day along with the five cold-pressed juices I planned on drinking.

The daily smoothie consisted of berries, coconut oil, almond milk, and a tiny bit of plant-based protein powder. Even though the energy it gave me is probably the only reason I survived the cleanse as well as I did, I cursed that smoothie every day for not being "pure" enough and for having what I viewed as too many calories. Also, the juice bar I was getting the juices and smoothie from every day had countless smoothie options on their menu, but once I started the cleanse with this particular one, called "Fountain of Youth," I was much too terrified to switch it up for fear that a different smoothie would throw off my entire cleansing mojo.

I usually stuck with drinking four green juices and one citrus and beet juice per day. I capped off each evening with my absolutely glorified vanilla almond milk treat. It was a small bottle of blended dehydrated almonds, coconut water, vanilla bean, and cinnamon, and to say I was living and breathing for drinking it each night would be an understatement. I went to bed dreaming about it and woke up the next day obsessing over how many hours it would be until I got to drink it again. I avoided going anywhere between the hours of 7 p.m. and 9 p.m. because I lived in dread of not being able to drink it chilled straight out of the refrigerator—how it tasted its best.

The *worst* was when I would bring the vanilla almond milk to class at night or to a restaurant where I was meeting friends and someone would ask me for a sip. I mean, how dare they . . . right? This was the only fuel I had to look forward to all day, save for the smoothie, of course, but I hated myself a little while I drank the smoothie, so the almond milk signified my truest happy moment of the day. It also came at the end of the day, when I was usually starving to the point of shakiness, so sipping on it was extra gratifying.

If people wanted to try the drink, I let them, but you better believe I calculated their one sip into the .00001 fewer calories I would be having in my day and tallied it in my brain as an *extra* exercise of my willpower. Being so empty made me feel so strong, and it's because all I cared about was that light, settled, and calm feeling in my stomach. If I could achieve that pure feeling, then all would be right in the world and I could go on with my life. I very much believed avoiding food in favor of cleansing would be my one and only shortcut to achieving that sensation as much as possible.

Also, at this point in my life and in my veganism, I was downright terrified about what was going to come next. I was in grad school for creative writing, but I knew in my heart that I wanted to leave my program and focus on the blog full-time. I was having issues with my vegan lifestyle and my relationship with food in general, and each day it was becoming clearer and clearer that what was going on with my family was very real and not something I could just shrug off. The combination of the two was wearing me thin, and I knew I needed to take action to get out of the dark gloom I was feeling.

The anger I felt toward the man who scammed my dad coupled with my hyperconcern about the legal battles surrounding the case were enough to send my entire being into panic overdrive. At the same time, having my life turned upside down put me in a place where, for the first time ever, I had to take a good, hard look at my life and ask myself what the hell I was doing and how on earth I was going to make this blogging business work if I really wanted it to.

Admitting to myself that the financial security of my family had been playing a huge role in the lifestyle I chose was tough. I had leaped into graduate school directly out of undergrad to pursue an MFA in creative writing, and I was living in a great neighborhood, working on a novel, and building my blog. I fear writing this and putting it out into the world even now because it's untrue that I didn't work extremely hard to make the blog successful, but the support of my parents and their guidance certainly helped a lot.

I knew I was working hard, and even when I offered to leave New York and come back to Northern California to work and save money on rent, my parents told me I was crazy. They wanted me to finish what I had started, and they wanted every door to be open to make sure I could do what I loved.

I knew exactly what they meant, but I couldn't shake the terrible feeling that maybe my living in New York and being in grad school was all wrong. Maybe I was just doing it because it was the next step I'd been planning for years. Maybe I was scared of what was out there beyond "the plan," and by working tirelessly to make the novel happen and throwing myself into school and classes and projects and essays, I was closing myself off from the opportunity to grow organically with life—to just be, and to create something for myself instead of take something that had been given to me.

I saw that nearly everyone else in my grad school program was a good five to ten years older than me. I listened to their stories of working in the gritty New York publishing industry and working their way up the totem pole to save enough money to come back to school. I sat silently in class while my classmates raged in debates over whether author Maggie Nelson's *Bluets* was a lyrical commentary on human suffering or a painful exploration of her own divorce. I cared about the work we were doing in school, but it was clear to me that I didn't care as *much* as I should—not as much as everyone else seemed to.

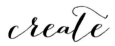

"MAYBE I WAS SCARED OF WHAT WAS OUT THERE BEYOND 'THE PLAN,' AND BY WORKING TIRELESSLY TO MAKE THE NOVEL HAPPEN AND THROWING MYSELF INTO SCHOOL AND CLASSES AND PROJECTS AND ESSAYS, I WAS CLOSING MYSELF OFF FROM THE OPPORTUNITY TO GROW ORGANICALLY WITH LIFE—TO JUST BE, AND TO CREATE SOMETHING FOR MYSELF INSTEAD OF TAKE SOMETHING THAT HAD BEEN GIVEN TO ME."

A Change of Heart

What I cared about was suddenly becoming painfully clear. I wanted to turn the blog into a business. Nothing in my life made as much sense as the blog did, and the success I had experienced thus far, even doing it on the side, was undeniable. Not only did I love blogging and crave everything about it as a creative and social outlet, but really my motivation was beyond that. I wanted to make something of it; I *needed* to make something of it, to show my dad how grateful I was and always will be for his lifelong selflessness by making it on my own. I needed him to know that even though his world had been turned upside down and sometimes outrageously undeserved things happen, he had given me the tools to be my own person and to build something I believed in.

He had given me the opportunity to pursue my passions, and there was no way on earth or in hell I was going to let that go to waste. I knew I needed to find my health so my stomach issues and growing eating disorder would stop plaguing my life and distracting me from building my brand. But before that could even happen, I had to sit down and ask myself *what* my next step was going to be. What made me happy?

I already knew my blog made me happy. But what else? I had to really think about it. What I came up with was, more or less: connecting with my blog readers, helping them find healthier versions of themselves, writing a *lot*, yoga, fitness, health, and spending time with supportive people who bring only positivity to my life.

I had spent so many years surrounding myself with people who were fun to be with, but as a result of the excess stress in my life, I finally felt really ready and quite desperate to shed some of the mediocre friendships I still had. It was time to focus solely on the people who were truly *there*; the people who understood me just by the expression on my face, the people who knew that no matter what I'd been handed in life I was busting my ass to make something work; and the people who weren't looking to play the game of "let's get shitfaced at brunch and find hot guys to pay for it."

When you're going through something tough, relying on people who want nothing but the best for you is key. During the hardest months when I had just found out what was going on with my family and was beginning to realize I was suffering from food issues far beyond my sensitive stomach, the genuine love from my true friends shone through like you wouldn't believe. Alternately, my patience for people who were *not* around for the right reasons dwindled away until it was nonexistent. Getting rid of their negative energy was so extremely necessary, and although it was sometimes hard to let go, it was always very, very worth it. I needed to do it.

Once I became attuned to what I actually wanted, the things I was growing mildly sick of doing actually became unbearable. I was sick of missing my family and my nieces reaching a whole new stage of childhood every time I got to see them; sick of playing along in grad school and sticking it out just because I'd started it; and really effing sick of obsessing about every bite I put into my mouth.

At the beginning of the mess that exploded with my family life and my food habits, I was much too absorbed in the issues at hand to understand that my eating was in freakish disarray. Instead of dealing with my disordered eating, I shoved it on the back burner and continued my juice cleansing, believing it was no more extreme than going vegetarian or cutting out gluten for the month.

But the difference was, while I trucked along on my thirty-day cleanse and lived for that nighttime vanilla almond milk, internally things were a' brewing. Over the course of that month, I slowly but surely made up my mind that changes were in store for real-life Jordan. I started viewing my life as something totally in my control—not just a product of being a daughter, a friend, a sister, an aunt, or a student. I *existed* outside of my relationships, and my life was mine to build.

rely

"WHEN YOU'RE GOING THROUGH SOMETHING TOUGH, RELYING ON PEOPLE WHO WANT NOTHING BUT THE BEST FOR YOU IS KEY."

What was the first step? No more grad school. It's true that getting my master's was a dream since I was young, but while I was in the program my priorities shifted. Blogging became something I loved so much that writing for anything other than the blog felt like a chore. Also, once I really drew inward, I realized that being there and forcing myself to do work I wasn't wholly passionate about was stunting me from creating my own life and was an excuse to continue relying on other people to help me create my future. Last, being anywhere you aren't 100 percent happy and engaged is not good for the soul—and I was finally realizing it.

The second step was moving back to Los Angeles. This one is harder to explain because it doesn't draw from the same logic as my leaving graduate school. New York was a dreamland. It was bursting with energy, creativity, and interesting people and offered outlets for just about every single thing I loved. It was a home for me when what I wanted most in life was to get out of Los Angeles and create a life for myself that had nothing to do with college, and it was also a playground of inspiration for the blog and healthy living. Not to mention that I was living with my lifelong best friend and had never felt more at home in an apartment, despite the space itself being a comical level of minuscule.

Oh, and I had developed great friendships with super-cool people who I loved spending time with, and I was making a name for myself in the healthy living community in the city. But for some reason, moving back to Los Angeles just *felt right*. And over my dead body was I going to deny myself something that rang true loud and clear.

soul

"BEING ANYWHERE YOU AREN'T 100 PERCENT HAPPY AND ENGAGED IS NOT GOOD FOR THE SOUL—AND I WAS FINALLY REALIZING IT."

I had control over very few things during those months. I had signed a two-year lease on my NYC apartment and had barely been there for one year. My family was so far away, I felt sick for not being there to comfort them during this rocky time. My skin was straight-up orange from an overabundance of beta-carotene, and my hair was falling out in clumps. My body hurt from walking down the street with no energy in my system, and I woke up in the middle of the night with excruciating pain shooting through my thighs and calves from trying to do yoga and train for a half marathon with zero protein, iron, or B$_{12}$ in my body.

Envisioning my life in Los Angeles felt good. I could drive to Northern California to surprise my parents whenever I felt like it, I could hang out at my sister's with my nieces all the time, I would be closer to a lot of my friends, and I would be in the sun and outside in the fresh air working on the blog and collaborating with other people in the health world. Also, I had great memories of living in LA in years prior and having a healthy relationship with food, and that's something I was desperately seeking. I felt like if I could just get back to that sunshine city, my food anxieties would melt away. (Side note: I wish!)

In the back of my mind I knew, of course, that moving across the country might actually make things worse with my food issues before they got better, but I was willing to try anything. I thought maybe making the move would give me that feeling of what I was so clearly missing. I didn't realize at the time that what I was really missing was nourishment and a connection between my mind and my body.

Come April, I told The New School I was leaving, I broke the lease on the apartment I shared with Katie, and I had a place lined up to move into in LA in the middle of the summer. Life felt upside down, but I was going to do everything in my power to straighten it back out.

9

WHAT IS THE POINT?

I ended up breaking my thirty-day juice cleanse a few days early, but not without much regret, self-loathing, and intense fear of reintroducing solid food. First of all, I don't think anyone's body is designed to go weeks on end without solid food. Perhaps it works for some people for one very particular reason or another, but for the average, healthy, active, and young person, I see absolutely no reason to long-term restrict from solid food unless you are trying to torture yourself.

The first seven days or so of the cleanse went swimmingly. I was on a cleansing high, extremely proud of myself for dedicating a full month to drinking nutrient-rich veggie juices and internally relieved that I didn't have to worry about my digestion problems because there wouldn't be anything in my stomach to digest. And on top of it, my close friends and classmates were commenting on my rapid weight loss (yet again), so I did feel a bit like a super-self-controlled cleansing rock star.

One Monday night on the second week of the cleanse, I threw on a black cropped sweater and a pair of tight, gray, wool pajama pants that I normally only wore to bed, and damn, did I feel tiny. I wore the ensemble to my fiction workshop class that night, and the general consensus was, "Yep, you're definitely on a cleanse. You look so small!" I loved every last compliment, every last glance, and every last reassuring remark that what I was doing was making a difference.

It sounds so sick looking back on it, but the psychology goes back to how satisfying it felt to reflect on the outside how empty and light I felt on the inside. Being empty signified triumph, willpower, and determination. And by portraying that hard-earned reward with my outward appearance, I felt I actually had something to show for my insane dedication to living pure.

By the eighth day in, I started panicking about my family and Danielle coming into town. There was no way I was going to end my cleanse early, and I had no idea how we were going to do anything or how I would be able to convey the full beauty of New York to them if I had to stop every thirty minutes to pee (so much liquid!) and run back home every two hours to get my next juice—because God forbid I drink a juice that wasn't fresh out of the fridge.

I started prepping my mom before her visit to New York by telling her it would be easier on everyone to have me cleansing because that way we could go to any restaurant and I would just bring my juice along. Her answer, which I could have guessed because it was becoming the standard response to all of my declarations involving food, juicing, or veganism: "Whatever you think, Jordan." It was clear that she was concerned about my extreme choice, but we also both admitted that she had no idea what it felt like to suffer from stomach problems in the way I did.

People were afraid to mess with what I staunchly proclaimed to be my cure-all diet, and in the same vein, they were afraid to tell me that what I was doing wasn't entirely healthy anymore. I'm a stubborn person, and I've never been one to succumb to someone else's suggestions until I'm ready to make a change myself. Plus, with my extreme devotion to the plant-based lifestyle and the fact that my growing career now centered on it, the people in my life would be insulting my entire livelihood by questioning the root of my dietary choices. With the exception of a couple of friends who spent a lot of time around me during those months, I only made people aware of the positivity that the lifestyle brought me.

I focused on the positive side of veganism in my mind, too. I didn't allow myself to think negatively about it, constantly reminding myself how healthy it was to eat such an abundance of fruits and vegetables. My digestion problems were mostly better than they'd been when I was eating animal protein, I prioritized my health above everything else, I cooked at home a lot more because it was hard to eat out, I got to connect with a lot of awesome people in the health community because of my vegan blogging, and on and on. Plus, I was *thin* and "SO HEALTHY." I truly believed I was *enlightened* by my vegan diet and I was so much more knowledgeable about health than I was before I got into veganism. In my mind, there was no going back to my previous way of life, and I convinced myself that any obsessions and anxieties I felt about food were purely because veganism was not the norm and it was hard to be a vegan in everyday life.

I also believed that my personality had a lot to do with it. I couldn't remember a time I had been totally lax about food or alcohol, other than parts of my wild college years, and I supposed that going vegan just made me more aware of additives and sugars and antibiotics and hormones and trans fats and preservatives I had never *really* been comfortable with in the first place. I didn't view moving away from any of that as a bad thing, but I failed to recognize that what I was doing was so much deeper than rejecting all of the unhealthy puzzle pieces of the Standard American Diet. I rationalized my overly extreme elimination by reading everything I could get my hands on about how *terrible* all of these elements were and by looking in the mirror incessantly and reminding myself how far I'd come.

I did wish I wasn't so uptight about food and envied people terribly who could eat whatever they wanted and feel fine later. I started to become aware of how much time I spent obsessing about food, but I pretty much thought it was because I was cleansing and couldn't wait to eat real food again. In a way, I felt I didn't deserve to eat real food like the other people around me because my stomach digested food so poorly and made me feel awful after eating. I reasoned that I would rather be uncomfortable and starving than uncomfortable and full—or even uncomfortable and appropriately satisfied by food.

I also felt I didn't deserve to eat real food as much as other people because I knew I was developing a control issue. I wasn't sure I knew how to eat and satisfy my hunger anymore, and I was afraid that if I ate as much as I saw other people eating, I wouldn't be able to stop after restricting for so long. After so much restriction and weeks of juice alone, I only knew how to take a few bites of food to barely sustain myself or to go way overboard and eat everything on the plate in response to deprivation. The things I allowed myself to eat in high volumes were bananas, berries, kale, broccoli, carrots, and sweet potatoes. Sometimes I would eat a kale and berry salad the size of a monster truck, and then I would immediately feel the roughage seeping into my stomach lining, producing acid, bloating my stomach, and making me absolutely hate myself for overindulging.

I also occasionally ate a lot of dates at once, mainly because it was one of my only sources of sugar and I craved the energy it brought me. But I always painfully regretted doing so because of the natural sugar that dates are packed full of. Every time I overate, I felt so sick and upset with myself, the only answer was to skip the next meal and have a juice instead. And don't even get me started on my weeklong bout with the 80/10/10 diet. I tried it after the thirty-day cleanse in a last-ditch attempt to heal myself through plants.

80/10/10 is a diet where 80 percent of your calories come from carbs, 10 percent from fats, and 10 percent from protein. In a raw vegan's case, the carbs come from fruit, the fats from nuts and seeds, and the protein from veggies. People who eat this way are encouraged to eat upwards of three thousand calories a day in order to get enough nutrients into their body, which was a concept that absolutely baffled me. Here I was, starving myself on an eight-hundred-calorie-a-day juice cleanse, and these people were claiming to be healthier and leaner than ever while eating so much food. I wasn't exactly enamored by the diet, especially because eating that much food in one day kind of petrified me, but I was intrigued.

I spent nights on end awake until the sun came up watching 80/10/10 raw vegan YouTube channels. I pored over their "Before and After" stories, their how-tos, their recipe videos, their "What I Eat in a Day" posts, and, in most cases, their eating disorder recovery stories. I started seeing a pattern among so many of them, also known as "high-carb, low-fat" raw vegans— they had had some kind of health issue, usually an eating disorder, and they were able to heal themselves through their 80/10/10 diet. Filling their bodies with plants instead of unhealthy binges was their key to recovery and letting go of their food fears.

I knew before I even tried the diet that drinking a smoothie with eight bananas in it in one sitting would make me feel catatonically ill, but because I saw the diet working so well for other healthy people (on YouTube . . .), I thought maybe it could be my answer too. I was so desperate to feel better yet so committed to maintaining my veganism that the promise of being able to make a change within the vegan umbrella sounded comforting.

overindulging

"SOMETIMES I WOULD EAT A KALE AND BERRY SALAD THE SIZE OF A MONSTER TRUCK, AND THEN I WOULD IMMEDIATELY FEEL THE ROUGHAGE SEEPING INTO MY STOMACH LINING, PRODUCING ACID, BLOATING MY STOMACH, AND MAKING ME ABSOLUTELY HATE MYSELF FOR OVERINDULGING."

So I spent the last couple weeks of my liquid cleanse ogling over bananas, apples, pears, and berries sold in abundance on NYC street corners. Virtually everything in the produce aisle at Whole Foods became literal food porn for my eyeballs and my stomach. You don't even want to know how much time I spent wandering around Whole Foods and other natural markets just for the sake of being surrounded by healthy food.

A Step Forward

The first day I broke my long-term liquid cleanse was absolutely terrifying. I wasn't fully through the thirty days yet, but something came over me one morning and I knew there was no way in hell I was going to continue starving myself. I had been lying on the couch in our apartment trying to work on the blog and my schoolwork, but the ultimate brain fog had washed over me. I was dizzy, fatigued, crampy, and downright obsessive about scrolling through photos of food I would never allow myself to eat. *All* I could think about was that damn vanilla almond milk I wouldn't be able to drink for another seven hours at least, and the thought of cracking open another green juice to sip on until my next two-hour mark made me nauseous.

I had just started drinking my Fountain of Youth smoothie, my midday sustenance, and I knew in my heart it just was not going to cut it. The protein powder in the smoothie was the most energizing part of my day hands down, and I figured if I could just have a little more of that, maybe I'd be fine. So I dug into my huge stash of plant-based protein powders, picked my favorite chocolate variation, and scooped out a big spoonful. (Side note: When I was in the middle of my extreme restriction, I would get ravenous cravings for *scoops* of protein powder. Alone. I wanted that powder in my system in all its chalky, crumbly, powdered glory. I usually reasoned with myself to add a few spoonfuls into a smoothie or an acai bowl rather than digging it straight out of the tub, but those cravings were so strong, I can feel their intensity in my core to this day.)

I was desperate to inhale the smoothie and far too concerned that if I poured it into my blender to mix with protein powder, I would lose some of the liquid by not being able to scrape it all back out again, so I frantically mixed the powder in with a spoon. The first sip was heavenly, but upon that very first taste I knew it wasn't going to be enough to sustain me. I added a scoop of almond butter, mixed it in, chugged the whole thing, and mentally decided that I was *for sure* going to eat solid food for dinner.

Once I let myself stray from the cleanse even the tiniest bit, I knew there was no going back. I had broken the mental challenge of it, and for me, the mental aspect was everything. If I could add protein powder to my smoothie, then mentally I could allow myself to eat vegetables. I had unleashed the rational side of my brain that knew there was *no* way two scoops of protein powder and a tablespoon (16 g) of almond butter would satisfy what I needed. I was empty, in every single way. Health food and control were not the answer, and cleansing certainly was not either.

The thought of eating real food again was both enticing and terrifying. To deal with the anxiety it gave me, I decided to run out to the store and buy a ton of bananas so I could start the 80/10/10 diet right away. When Katie came home from work that evening and saw the mountain of bananas spilling over the counter of our teeny-tiny kitchen, her reaction was, "I'm not even going to ask."

Her boyfriend came over later and actually laughed out loud about how many bananas I had bought. It looked like a scene out of a hoarders documentary. And in truth I felt like more of a normal eater than I had in weeks because at least now I was open to the idea of eating solid food, which made me a little more socially acceptable . . . right?

Right?! (Kidding.)

And quickly, on the topic of boyfriends: I most definitely, 100 percent did not have one throughout the depths of my eating disorder. When I briefly dated people in New York, my food preferences were the main topic of our discussions and eventually became such a big barrier between us, the relationship petered out before it even began. Also, because of the anxiety

empty

"I WAS EMPTY, IN EVERY SINGLE WAY. HEALTH FOOD AND CONTROL WERE NOT THE ANSWER, AND CLEANSING CERTAINLY WAS NOT EITHER."

I was dealing with and the major dedication to the blog and my healthy lifestyle, the people I was interested in were typically just as unavailable as I was. I'm grateful that I was single for this period of my life because involving someone else in the mess that was my mind space would only have caused more difficulty.

And even though my anxiety issues were not disguisable, one thing I was able to hide was just how bad my eating disorder was becoming. When my mom and sister visited, two people who know me extremely well, they only got a glimpse into how bad it was. They noticed I had become more anxious about food and even pickier and stricter with my choices, but they didn't see how much I was suffering on the inside. No one did, because I would barely even admit it to myself!

After my trial and error with the 80/10/10 diet—all you need to know is that I ate so many bananas on the diet I thought I would never be able to walk again, and it left me with the most ravenous sugar cravings I've ever experienced—I felt like it was time to go back to square one. Every time I dedicated myself to making a dietary change like that, I called it going "back to the basics." I would have a green smoothie for breakfast, a kale salad with berries for lunch, and roasted veggies with quinoa drizzled in fresh lemon juice for dinner, with few to no exceptions. Even though this was a manageable, clean, healthful way of eating during my first plant-based cleanse, after living that way for over a year and a half, my body was yearning for more, and certainly for far more variation.

single

"I'M GRATEFUL THAT I WAS SINGLE FOR THIS PERIOD OF MY LIFE, BECAUSE INVOLVING SOMEONE ELSE IN THE MESS THAT WAS MY MIND SPACE WOULD ONLY HAVE CAUSED MORE DIFFICULTY."

The 80/10/10 Diet

A note about the 80/10/10 diet: I am not knocking it for anyone who feels it works for them. The beauty of listening to our bodies is that we are all so entirely different, and we all have to find what works best for us. I understand I didn't eat that way for very long, but it was long enough for my body to tell me it didn't work for me and definitely wouldn't have made me feel well long-term. I wouldn't advise it for those of us who are prone to extremes, but if you have found solace in eating that way and feel sustained, then I support you for listening to your body!

I started thinking again about how nice it might be and how much energy it might give me to reintroduce eggs and fish into my diet, and every time I did, my mind went directly back to what Jillian had said to me in the car nearly a year before: "If you like fish, why deprive yourself?" Basically, the gist of what she was saying, and the core point I hung on to, was, What's the point? *What is the goddamn point*, if you're starving yourself and feeling terrible and weak and unhealthy and bloated and depressed and obsessive? What. Is. The. Point.

However, I was still getting ahead of myself. First I had to try fish and see if it was even something I enjoyed and wanted to continue eating. I was semi-hopeful that the experience would go awry, and I would be able to repledge myself to veganism and the plant-based lifestyle with a vengeance. Except I think I knew somewhere inside that that would not be the case, and that's why my mind was already running rampant with concerns about what would come next. My body was so ready for more sustenance. Despite the part of me that was terrified, I was also intensely relieved. I might actually be moving toward remedying my stomach problems and severe compulsions, and that gave me enough hope to hang on to.

10

THE WAKE-UP CALLS

Once I got the "What is the point?" mentality into my mind, it was only a matter of time before I realized what I needed to do for myself. It was finally starting to soak in that there *was* no longer a point. There was absolutely no reason to continue my cycle of deprivation and obsession and eventually complete isolation from people I loved who were very worried about me.

The tipping point was simply a culmination of months of difficulty tied in with particular events, usually where food was involved, that left me feeling so incredibly different and removed from who I was once was. That and my health, of course. Health was still a priority and something I was passionate about, even though I had lost sight of it in my desire to be as pure and clean as possible. Once my body started showing signs of unhealthiness, I knew some changes had to be made.

For one, my skin had taken on an awkward shade of orange that contrasted with an overall face and chest blotchiness I had developed from nutrient deficiencies. The beta-carotene from my sweet potato and carrot "safe foods" had taken over my pallid East Coast postwinter skin tone, and my teeth were losing the bright white quality they'd always had because of the overabundant green juices and smoothies I was drinking. My hair was thinning, refused to grow, and on more than one occasion, slipped out of my scalp in a noticeably large clump while I was showering. Not cool.

On top of the outward physical signs, my body was rebelling in other ways. I had lost my period in the early months of 2014, and at first I didn't think that much of it. I wasn't on birth control anymore, so my body wasn't relying on anything external to regulate my cycle. I had an inkling that my diet played some kind of hand in the loss of my period, but it took me several months to even realize my body was crying for help. In a twisted way, I *liked* not having to deal with it every month, and I tried everything in my power to convince myself it was not my body's response to a lack of nutrients.

Another part of me felt that the loss of my period couldn't be a *huge* issue, because it's a problem I generally associated with people who are significantly undernourished. What I didn't realize was that although I was not sickly thin, I was undernourished. It was confusing to me because although I was thin for my frame, I hadn't dipped down to an all-time low or unhealthy weight. I looked like someone who ate well and worked out frequently. I still had curves, and while the five- to ten-pound (2.3 to 4.5 g) fluctuations that occurred between juice cleanses affected my image of my own body down to my very core, I knew they weren't extremely noticeable on the outside. Yes, people noticed and commented and took extra-long sideways glances now and again if they really knew me, but it had been months and months since someone told me I was looking too thin.

That's another reason why I let my food anxieties take over my life in such a strong way. I didn't look unhealthy. I was not skeletal. You had to know me well or have a very clear understanding of how nutrition affects the body to see I had deficiencies. My family could tell because they know what a healthy Jordan looks like and how much I had deviated from that. Nutritionists and eating disorder therapists could tell because they know what signs to look for with food obsessions and anxieties, and I was exhibiting quite a few of them. Extremely perceptive individuals could tell because after a few minutes in conversation with me, it was clear that my mind was wrapped up in a jumbled web of disordered-eating obsessions and compulsions.

A Crucial Conversation

Jamie Graber, a close friend of mine and owner of an organic raw vegan restaurant in New York, recognized it because she had been in a similar position, and for that I am eternally grateful. Jamie and I were meeting one afternoon along with another friend of ours to plan an event at her restaurant. I was inviting my blog readers, and it was going to be a meet-and-greet type of event with delicious organic food from her restaurant.

After we hammered out the details of the event, Jamie asked me about my vegan diet out of her own curiosity. At the time, we didn't know each other well, and being a fountain of knowledge about all things raw vegan, she wanted to know more about where my food choices stemmed from. I told her about my journey from stomach problems to vegetarian-ish to vegan and so on, and she listened intently.

Then, out of nowhere, she asked me if I menstruated regularly. My answer was, of course, no, because it had been months since I'd had my period, but other than brief mentions here and there to my mom and Katie, I hadn't actually admitted it out loud or thought about the health repercussions.

The concern on her face when I said I hadn't had a period in six months hit me hard, kind of like waking up from a long, confused slumber. Why had I been blinding myself for so long? I prided myself on prioritizing health and was doing everything in my power to live as purely as possible, yet here I was ignoring a huge sign from my body. Jamie suggested trying to eat a piece of freshwater fish each week to get some vitamin B_{12} into my system and hopefully regulate my cycle.

I was astounded. Fish?! That would mean breaking veganism. I wasn't sure I had it in me to make a change so radical. I could hardly bring myself to eat a bowl of black beans and quinoa for the sake of having protein in my system, let alone branch out and put animal flesh in my body for the first time in so long. But at the same time, it sounded so satisfying, and I started imagining what it might be like to eat a meal and feel satiated afterward. It also sounded easier on my poor, tattered digestive system than some of the roughage-heavy salads and raw vegan nut and seed concoctions I was eating with abandon. And needless, to say it sounded more desirable than another freaking ten-banana smoothie.

She also suggested getting weekly B$_{12}$ shots as an alternative, but going to the doctor every week to get a supplement shot into my bloodstream sounded so far removed from who I was and who I wanted to be. I wanted food to heal me. I wanted it to fuel me and sustain me, and I wanted it to not wreak havoc on my body but instead to make me the healthiest I could be *naturally*. I thought that's what I had been doing all along, but my body had changed, and I wasn't allowing myself to listen to it.

Perhaps that was the most frustrating part of the whole journey. I was bending over backward, making excuses, shielding myself from life, killing myself on the inside with each and every starvation-induced thought and obsession, and for what? To hurt my body and strip myself of adequate nutrients to thrive and to feel good? To stay awake throughout the night panicking about what breakfast might look like in the morning, how many ounces of a pound (grams of a kilogram) it would make me gain, how much I would have to exercise to burn it off, how tired I was going to be after exercising and not sleeping or eating properly, and how I was possibly going to navigate my work and social life while shoving my food demons further and further into the back of my mind?

Yeah, that sounds like hell to me. The world was inedible, and I was now realizing it. The recognition of how much I was truly suffering was creeping over me and sinking into my bones and blood and mind and heart the way things always seem to do with me—long overdue but stronger than ever.

listen

"I WANTED FOOD TO HEAL ME. I WANTED IT TO FUEL ME AND SUSTAIN ME, AND I WANTED IT TO NOT WREAK HAVOC ON MY BODY BUT INSTEAD TO MAKE ME THE HEALTHIEST I COULD BE *NATURALLY*. I THOUGHT THAT'S WHAT I HAD BEEN DOING ALL ALONG, BUT MY BODY HAD CHANGED, AND I WASN'T ALLOWING MYSELF TO LISTEN TO IT."

So strong, in fact, I wasn't sure I could wait another waking hour before eating the damn piece of fish, even though another part of me was petrified and unsure that I would be able to eat it once it was in front of me.

On the long, muggy walk home from the East Village to the West Village that afternoon, I tossed over a trillion options and questions in my mind. I *could* try the fish, but where on earth would I get it? How could I trust that it wouldn't contain hormones and fillers to make it bigger or taste better? How would I know it was fresh? What if the natural oil from the fish sent my stomach into a greasy, oily, lubricated, painful-bloating-sickening overload and I gained ten pounds (4.5 kg) on the spot or felt so ill I couldn't move?

Above all, the biggest question in my mind was, *What* would people think if they knew that The Blonde Vegan was eating fish? It wasn't necessarily the fear of other people's judgment that petrified me (although that was scary too), but the fact that I would be going against the word I had so faithfully and loyally been advocating. I told people that veganism was the answer to my lifelong digestion problems, I recommended it to people who were suffering as I had been, and I coached hundreds of my readers through weekly plant-based cleanse programs to lose weight and find their health and happiness. Everything I stood for was rooted in a plant-based lifestyle. How could I eat fish and still be that person?

Furthermore, I had fully decided to leave graduate school to pursue the blog full-time. I now depended on the blog for income in a way I hadn't when I was in school. Without my blog's success, I would have to reevaluate my life yet again, just when I thought I had found what truly made me happy. And blogging *did* make me happy—I didn't want to give it up, and it didn't seem fair or rational that a bite of fish should have any hand in tarnishing the brand I had worked so hard to build.

Would I lose my entire following and have to create a new blog? What would it be about? Couldn't I just switch my label from "plant-based vegan" to "plant-based vegan plus fish" and call it a day? People would have to understand . . . right? And then there was the option to eat fish every so often in private to up my B_{12} level, but the thought of introducing non-vegan food into my diet and not being truthful about it on the blog made me extremely uncomfortable. My readers came to me with their digestion problems and health issues, and for me to sit there and tell them that veganism worked for me when it didn't anymore would just be wrong.

At that point I was still getting ahead of myself by worrying. First I had to do the hard part: I had to try the fish and see if it was even something I enjoyed and wanted to continue eating. Worrying gave me something to hold on to that distracted me from the problem at hand, but after that conversation with Jamie, I knew I needed to address the problem and actually step outside my comfort zone. In order to do that, I needed to try the fish—scary!

I picked up a piece of salmon on my way home from the East Village—I told you I don't mess around once I make up my mind—from a macrobiotic restaurant called Souen. I had eaten there dozens of times, and the only non-vegan item on their menu was freshwater fish. Even Jamie had suggested it to me and said she trusted it. I felt pretty hopeless and panicked in the non-vegan world, so her word meant a lot.

At this point, the very few people who had an idea of my inner tumult could not have been entirely surprised that I was about to try fish. Those two people were Katie, who not only saw me every day but shared a small living space with me, and my mom, who was on the other side of the country but knows me so well there is no hiding anything from her. Because of their involvement with my diminishing state of being due to food, it was only fitting that I send both of them a photo of the miniature salmon fillet sitting, simmering, and steaming on my plate and filling my apartment with an aroma I hadn't known for years. When other people had eaten fish around me, I'd blocked out the sights and smells because it was so off-limits in my mind.

blogging

"AND BLOGGING *DID* MAKE ME HAPPY—I DIDN'T WANT TO GIVE IT UP, AND IT DIDN'T SEEM FAIR OR RATIONAL THAT A BITE OF FISH SHOULD HAVE ANY HAND IN TARNISHING THE BRAND I HAD WORKED SO HARD TO BUILD."

So before I dove in, I snapped a photo and sent it off. I was used to photographing my every meal by now. I had been blogging about my meals every day for nearly a year, but taking a picture of *animal protein* that was about to go into *my body* felt so foreign. I think a part of me needed to send it to them to make the whole situation feel more real, more tangible, like something I could hold on to and categorize as truth instead of some crazy split-second decision that would derail my lifestyle.

I also must have been proud somewhere inside because sending off the photo felt a bit like sending a picture of a good report card or a first-day-of-school snapshot. I knew both my mom and Katie would be flooded with shock, relief, and confusion, and they would congratulate me on moving so far out of my comfort zone. So maybe it was more like sending them a picture of me skydiving or paragliding over the mountains—something extreme and wild and so distant from the person I had been for so long but so close I could taste it (literally) at the same time.

When I say my salmon fillet was miniature, I mean it literally. It was pounded thin by the restaurant and sliced jagged on its side, like perhaps there was hardly enough to go around and fill all the orders that day. I didn't mind; I couldn't even conceive of having a fuller plate of salmon in front of me, and it was only later when I looked back on that photo that I saw how tiny it really was. A thin, flaky piece of pink fish, juicy and tempting, giving me a writhing panic attack and a thrill all at once. One tiny piece of fish served as the barrier between my unswaying vegan label and what inevitably existed on the other side.

When I finally worked up the courage to taste it, the warmth and texture of the fish filled me with unearthly surprise and pleasure. It tasted good, sure, but it was beyond that. I was eating something that was not only "solid food," but was full of vitamins and minerals my body was absolutely desperate for, something that could only be described as the *medicine* I needed to heal the damage I had been doing to myself.

And no, I was not so lost in my illness to believe that one piece of fish would cure several years' worth of vitamin and mineral deficiencies. But damn, did it feel good to eat the salmon and prove to myself that not only was I capable of making a change and listening to my body, I was capable of satiating myself and knowing it wouldn't kill me. It wouldn't even hurt me. Nor would it bring my worst fears to life, the ones rooted in stomach pain, bloat, weight gain, heartburn, acid reflux, and painful intestinal reactions to animal protein after not having it for so long. I felt fine! Hell, I even felt kind of . . . normal—a bit unbalanced and panicked about what my next meal or next *meals* would look like, but a little freaking normal nonetheless.

By the time I finished, I had to report back to Katie and my mom to continue making the situation feel real. If I didn't, I worried I would just start to see it as a bump in the road and quietly return to my strict veganism and juice cleansing. "OMG it was so good!!!" I typed. "I BET!" my mom responded, and "I can't believe this! I'm so proud of you!" Katie said.

It almost sounds silly, two grown women congratulating another grown woman on eating food that satiates her, but if only I could convey to you how badly I needed to hear it. And that fish experience, along with their words of encouragement, was the tip of the iceberg in my wake-up calls. I was already making up my mind that I was going to be "vegan plus fish," and maybe, just maybe, vegan plus fish and eggs if I tried eggs and found them satisfying and okay with my system.

That way I could come out to my readers in what felt like a more under-standable way. "Hey guys, don't worry, I'm still basically vegan, I just need to eat fish once in a while so my body can function properly. UGH, bodies always needing shit, you understand???" I envisioned it over and over: how I would do it, what I would say, and how they would react. I knew I would lose the diehards, the ethical vegans that already despised me because I ate honey on a vegan diet (and I know what they're thinking right now: You were never "VEGAN" because you ate honey, you liar! *I get it, trust me*), but I was fine with that. I knew there were enough supporters to outweigh the anger that was to come and the readers I would lose.

satiate

"IT ALMOST SOUNDS SILLY, TWO GROWN WOMEN CONGRATULATING ANOTHER GROWN WOMAN ON EATING FOOD THAT SATIATES HER, BUT IF ONLY I COULD CONVEY TO YOU HOW BADLY I NEEDED TO HEAR IT."

While I waited to come forward with my changes and decide what my new diet would look like, the next wake-up call came. This one was a bit more startling and altogether harder to accept than the careful reintroduction of salmon. This one was messier because it dealt with the actual, deep-rooted problem. It was the reason why the salmon was so petrifying to me: the nasty, dirty, unkempt back room of the pretty vegan storefront I had been keeping, sweeping, maintaining, and displaying for so long. It was the pain that existed inside the health-conscious shell I had created, the exterior that defined me.

Identifying the Problem

To be completely honest, I'm not sure how, when, or if the truth of the pain would have struck me if I hadn't had a life-changing conversation with one of my closest friends, Tara, over dinner in midtown one night. I had met Tara through health blogging when I first moved to New York. We met on Instagram when she reached out to me, "@SkinnybyTara," (now @TheWholeTara) by writing on one of my "@theblondevegan" photos and saying, "You live in NY?! Why aren't we friends?!?!"

Our friendship was easy and quick to develop. We bonded over yoga, health food, juicing, being sunshine state transplants in the big city (she was born and raised in Miami), and the fact that we were both brand new to health-blogging success. That night Tara and I both ordered kale salads, hers with egg whites, mine without. When she ordered the egg whites, she turned and said, "I'm having a non-vegan night, I know."

This struck me because Tara had never really *called* herself a vegan. She wasn't stuck in the label like I was, and even though she was basically vegan and ate very similar to the way I did, I was surprised that she nearly apologized for the egg whites. I quickly told her I was experimenting with eggs and fish too, as of earlier that week, and I think she was partially blown away and partially not surprised at all—considering she knew I had been searching for balance and my stomach problems had been expecially bad lately.

Then we got onto a topic I will never forget. It kind of came flooding out all at once, on both our parts, that we had been silently suffering for quite some time. Tara shared with me that she had been going through some food struggles, and in listening to her story, it suddenly became scintillatingly clear to me for the first time: I had an eating disorder. Not a cutesy, "Oh, I'm kind of afraid to eat other foods because I've been vegan for so long" issue with food, but a full-blown, mind-numbing, anxiety-pulsating "I will use food, or the lack thereof, to cure anything and everything about my life" kind of eating disorder.

Eating disorder. Disordered eating. Habits of disordered eating. Eating disorder tendencies. A tendency and habits toward eating in a disorderly way. The term sounds so extreme, but all at once it hit me and I knew—that's what was inside me, that's what was hurting me so much, that's what I was suffering from, and maybe I had been suffering from it all along.

Maybe the little girl who stood in front of the pantry at age eleven and swore to herself she would never touch junk food again, when she meant it with all her heart, when she carried it out for days and weeks at a time, and when she felt miserable, sick, and like a failure when she couldn't keep it up—maybe she had been suffering too. Maybe the five-year-old, the adolescent, and the young adult me who had been reprimanded and watched, watched, always watched, by well-meaning loved ones for eating too much of the foods that were sure to bother her tummy, maybe she was harboring more pain and frustration inside than she could have known.

suffering

"THE TERM SOUNDS SO EXTREME, BUT ALL AT ONCE IT HIT ME AND I KNEW—THAT'S WHAT WAS INSIDE ME, THAT'S WHAT WAS HURTING ME SO MUCH, THAT'S WHAT I WAS SUFFERING FROM, AND MAYBE I HAD BEEN SUFFERING FROM IT ALL ALONG."

Maybe when foods became "off-limits" the moment I associated them with stomach problems, back when I was too young to even *know* that food and weight had anything to do with one another, I learned to associate food with failure and success. The more I could keep off-limits foods out of my life, the stronger I felt. When the scale went down, I got more compliments, more praise for "listening to my body," and, for a while, less stomach pain. But it always came back, and with it came a sense of dread and guilt and sadness that no food or avoidance of it could remedy.

My life had become a yo-yo. A juice cleanse to shed the weight, the guilt, the sadness, and the anxiety would be followed by excess, albeit exceptionally healthy, food to fill the massive, gaping hole in my stomach where balance, confidence, and contentment should have been. I had also toyed with my blood sugar so much, it was a wonder I could still see results from cleansing and eating so minimally.

I came out and said it in my conversation with Tara that night, and it was like finally realizing, after years of pain and sickness, that I had the flu and needed to rest to get better or like yearning for something I couldn't put my finger on and then realizing I'd found exactly what I needed to satisfy it. It was relief, pure and simple, in its plainest form. And just like I needed to take photos of my salmon and send them to Katie and my mom to make eating it feel real, asserting my realization aloud to Tara over and over again made it feel not only more real but somehow more manageable.

dread

"BUT IT ALWAYS CAME BACK, AND WITH IT CAME A SENSE OF DREAD AND GUILT AND SADNESS THAT NO FOOD OR AVOIDANCE OF IT COULD REMEDY."

I had an eating disorder. I was going to fix it. I had made choices, done things to the extreme, and created a life in which my eating disorder was the norm. It was a part of me, masked as something else. Something far more socially acceptable—admirable, even. Something beyond the boundaries of plant-based vegan food blogger and passionate health foodie, although those were nice descriptions I also fell into, and they made my life and my obsessions far easier to explain. I had now gone beyond those margins, and the labels were just shielding me from what I had truly turned into.

At dinner Tara and I discussed my brand-new semblance of a plan of attack. Who was I going to tell first? Would I write about it on the blog? How was I going to get help? Would I move away from veganism entirely? These questions were all swimming wildly in my mind, but I knew the first thing I needed to do was call my mom. I was terrified and exhilarated all at once, feeling like she probably had an idea this was coming but also wondering if she might be shocked or even disagree with me about how bad it had gotten.

When I called her on my long walk home from the restaurant, I began the conversation as I always do when I'm hopelessly nervous about something—by rambling like a psychopath. How my day was, how the blog was doing, how school was, the weather, my friends, and, oh yeah, I just finished dinner with Tara and we talked about some heavy stuff and I am pretty sure I have an eating disorder. I winced, picking up my pace and half-stomping, half-leaping over the city subway vents like it was my job.

"Yeah, I think you do too," she said back. WHAT? She knew?! How did she know and not say anything?

"Wait, you really think so?" I asked, dumbfounded and freakishly relieved at the same time.

"Yes, absolutely."

Well, wow. Apparently she had been questioning my rising food anxieties on her own terms and was waiting for me to realize it on my own, which I very much understand on her part because with something as sensitive and intricately wound as an eating disorder, there aren't many ways to bring it up without totally offending and pushing away the sufferer.

We talked long and hard and deep about everything I was feeling, everything she had noticed food-wise and obsession-wise the last few times she had been with me, and how she observed that it had gotten particularly bad in the last few months. She knew I was cleansing more often; that my already severe food limitations had basically quadrupled; and that, well, I didn't look like the healthy, happy, thriving daughter she had always known me to be.

I assured her I would do everything I could to find the best eating disorder therapist and nutritionist New York had to offer, even though I was moving back to Los Angeles in a matter of two months and I knew my work with the specialists would only just be beginning. I didn't want to wait. I didn't want to continue living in the prison that was my mind when it came to food. I wanted out, and for the first time in nearly two years I had an idea of what *getting out* would entail.

11

GETTING HELP & COMING CLEAN

Getting help was extremely tricky to navigate. I knew that guidance and advice from both an eating disorder therapist and an eating disorder nutritionist were a must, but I also knew that most of the work was going to consist of me rewiring my mindset about my lifelong relationship with food.

My extreme relationship with food was an addiction, whether it matches up with traditional definitions of addiction diseases or not. Food was an obsession for me, just as the intense avoidance of certain foods was an obsession. The more I emphasized food avoidance, the more I obsessed over food. The more I gave in and let myself eat what I wanted, the more guilt I developed and yet again the more obsessed I got with "starting fresh" with plant-based food or cleansing each and every day.

The addiction was a battle I had been fighting all my life: the push and pull of eating well versus eating the one little thing that tipped my stomach over the edge, the praise and the watchful eyes, and the mechanism of control when everything else was spiraling beyond my reach. What my veganism had done was take the addiction to a whole new level. I finally had a way to *describe* my food avoidances and health prioritizations. If I used the term *vegan*, or better yet, *plant-based vegan*, to describe my diet and lifestyle, people cut me some slack. They either didn't understand exactly what it meant, so they let me do my thing, or they totally understood and helped me cater to it.

Instead of feeling judged and misunderstood, I felt I was accepted because I had made a choice that had a name. I had a label that felt very safe and cozy, and even if people continued to misunderstand it, they had no choice but to deal with it. It's not like being on a label-free healthy diet and refusing fries or a drink out at a bar and having to deal with peers who try to get you to just have it anyway. Plant-based veganism takes it a step further. It was my *lifestyle*, and even though there was still pressure from others to "let loose," I learned early on that people were much more likely to understand my choices once they had a label to grasp on to.

Without the outside chatter and the noise and the constant "No thanks, I'm good," assertions and the sideways looks and, most of all, the overin-dulgences I associated with not being vegan, I felt *safe*. I felt like at the end of the day, no matter what went wrong, even if I overate or got into an argu-ment or my life as I knew it was crumbling apart, at least I was a goddamn vegan. I was healthy, and I was making the choice to eat clean and pure and stick to it every single day. Veganism was consistent in my life. It was reliable. My green juices were my refuge; in some way, it is still hard for me to understand why they meant so much to me, why I would trek 2 miles (3 k) in the snow for the perfect juice, yet the attachment is so clear at the same time. They made me feel mentally strong when my insides were weaker than weak.

In the early days of recovery with my eating disorder therapist, I realized I was overwhelmed with emotion about everything and controlling my food, and therefore my body and what felt like my mind, was my out. I knew I was a tightly wound person. I knew I had inherited my dad's OCD, my mom's sensitivity, and both of my parents' innate ability to be incredibly hard on themselves, and I was simply carrying it out in a different way than I had seen them do for all the years of my existence.

And then there was the whole food anxiety thing. If I was scared of greasy foods at the ages of five and six, imagine me thinking about trying them for the sake of my mental health after years of not going near them with a ten-foot pole. Imagine the girl who stopped eating red meat in high school as a control mechanism, nine years later, as a twenty-three-year-old, sitting in her therapist's office trying to explain *why* the thought of eating red meat was petrifying if not seemingly impossible.

I knew I didn't have to make any choices I didn't want to make, and I didn't have to let go of any labels I didn't want to lose. No one was forcing me to do anything. Even my nutritionist told me we could make a vegan diet work from there on out if it was important to me to remain that way. She did stress that it would be hard to get my blood sugar restabilized and to get my hormones back in check if I stuck to my rigid regimen of plants, but it could be done. I'm guessing I wasn't her first rodeo of the plant-based sort—which is why I think she was all the more stunned when I told her I didn't care to remain plant-based and she could put me on any meal plan she wanted.

"Well, this is going to be easier than I thought!" she said, her big, warm smile spreading across her face and highlighting her grandmotherly demeanor. She told me over and over again that I was going to be just fine and that I had already done so much of the mental work that can sometimes take months and years to accomplish. *But no*, I wanted to tell her. *Can't you see? I'm terrified. I still need so much help.*

I knew that letting go of the restrictions would only be a part of it. I saw her point, that my willingness to try new things was helpful to the process and set me apart from some of her more severe patients, but I still felt violently unstable in my footing. I wanted to let go of the restrictions because I knew they were ruining my life and deteriorating my health, but I was also petrified of letting them go. They had been my comfort for so long, my pacifier when things were going wrong. If my relationship with food was fine and dandy, where would I channel the sadness when it came to me?

refuge

"VEGANISM WAS CONSISTENT IN MY LIFE. IT WAS RELIABLE. MY GREEN JUICES WERE MY REFUGE . . . THEY MADE ME FEEL MENTALLY STRONG WHEN MY INSIDES WERE WEAKER THAN WEAK."

Friends and Family

I frequently mention how important the people in my life have been throughout my recovery process. Tommy is a godsend, and the fact that we understand each other on such a superhuman level is one of the most comforting feelings in the world. Each and every one of my friends, family, and readers have all found ways to be there for me, regardless of their ability to understand having an eating disorder in itself, and their support has been one of the main reasons I have progressed the way I have.

I tried to explain this newfound hesitation to my therapist, and she told me it was very normal to fear letting go of this unhealthy relationship I'd relied on for so long—even though it was a relationship with *food*, something I would have to deal with daily regardless of how I felt about it. She asked me to compare my fear of letting go to other parts of my life and see if perhaps *holding on*, especially when things got rough, was a pattern of mine. Umm, let's see here. Yes, and yes. Remember Tommy, the boy I told you about who was my first love and dear friend? We've remained close all these years; no matter what difficulties have come our way, we've held on—we are the same, in that way. That's yet another reason, I realized then, why he is so special to me. He understands my neurotic and obsessive mindset in a way that few other people have.

Then I started thinking about the obsessions in all areas of my life. There they were, loud and clear. The blog? I dove in, 100 percent dedicated, balls to the wall and ready to write and photograph new content every single day, engage with every single reader that came to the site, create products to sell, and connect, try as I might, with every other blogger who had inspired me. And that, I reasoned, was a very good side effect of my obsessive personality trait. Sometimes having an extreme means extremely good things can come from it, while other times the extreme is more negative—in which case, it's a force to be reckoned with.

What I had to learn to do, and continue to learn to this day, is distinguish the bad extremes from the good. And sometimes they aren't so black and white as the eating disorder and the blog. For instance, I am an extremely sensitive person. On the one hand, my sensitivity makes me extra compassionate to my friends, family, readers, and people I come across, and it allows me to connect quickly with them on a deeper level. I listen, I understand, and I can sympathize with them because even if I haven't been there, I know what it feels like to hurt.

That's the good side of it—lots of friends and the deep connections! I have many close, close friendships that sustain me and help make me who I am. On the other hand, my sensitivity can get in the way of my life sometimes. If I am in an argument with someone I love, it can bring me down all day to the point where I get nothing done and I ruminate and obsess over the conversation we had (or didn't have, in some cases) until the situation mends itself. Often I know that the issue in my mind was much, much larger of a deal than it was in reality. But because I am so extreme, because I am *wired* that way, I can't always reason with myself in the moment.

That has been the hardest part of my recovery process, hands down: determining whether an extreme is good or bad, right or wrong, worthy or unworthy of my attention. In eating disorder recovery, those extremes usually crop up in relation to food. I will get a massive craving for a brownie (non-vegan, refined sugar, full of ingredients I wouldn't have touched before) in the middle of the day, for example, and I don't know what the hell is going on. Do I listen to my body and indulge so I'll satisfy my craving,

friends

"THAT'S THE GOOD SIDE OF IT—LOTS OF FRIENDS AND THE DEEP CONNECTIONS! I HAVE MANY CLOSE, CLOSE FRIENDSHIPS THAT SUSTAIN ME AND HELP MAKE ME WHO I AM."

be proud of myself, and go on with my day? Or is that just my body telling me it *thinks* it wants sugar because it's obsessing over something it didn't have for so long?

It's *really* hard to distinguish between those two things, and sometimes there is no right answer at all. Sometimes I walk the line between avoiding the brownie at all costs and eating five brownies all in one sitting to stick it to the man. And then I feel sick and overly full and, my worst fears come to life, bloated and nauseated due to food. Learning to eat my once off-limits foods again *while* practicing moderation but not too much moderation to the point of restriction became one of the most difficult tasks in the world.

It seemed simple enough—just don't think too hard about what you're putting into your mouth. If you don't obsess, there will be far less of a chance that the food will upset your stomach in the way you imagine. If I could just learn to eat something without thinking about the end product of every calorie, imagining every last nutrient property of the food, basically swallowing its nutritional value label right along with the meal, then I knew my life would be a lot simpler.

And there was something else I knew I had to do right off the bat to simplify and get rid of my anxiety about being The Blonde Vegan who was no longer vegan. I had to come forward to my blog readers, and at the same time, pretty much anyone I've ever known in my life, about my dietary transition and thus, my eating disorder. I didn't have to write about my orthorexia on the blog, but I wanted to. It was a crucial part of why I stopped eating a

simpler

"IF I COULD JUST LEARN TO EAT SOMETHING WITHOUT THINKING ABOUT THE END PRODUCT OF EVERY CALORIE, IMAGINING EVERY LAST NUTRIENT PROPERTY OF THE FOOD, BASICALLY SWALLOWING ITS NUTRITIONAL VALUE LABEL RIGHT ALONG WITH THE MEAL, THEN I KNEW MY LIFE WOULD BE A LOT SIMPLER."

plant-based diet, and it was the main information I wanted to share with people who were also suffering. I knew I had to do it, I just didn't know how.

I wanted to wait until I knew exactly what my new diet would look like. What if I decided to eat predominantly plant-based in the end and I had to take it all back? Or what if I decided to eat beef *all the time* because it miraculously made me feel loads better and that needed to be an integral part of the "coming out" story? I knew there was no perfect moment, no surefire way to go about it and keep everyone's happiness intact, so I did what I do best . . .

I sat down on a park bench and I wrote—frantically. I wrote madly, without coming up for air, typing every last word of my journey in the "Notes" section of my phone until the battery was on 1 percent and then died. When it died, I wrote the rest in my head. I walked into a corner store and bought a pen and paper. I wrote and wrote, and then I wrote it all over again. The story came out exactly the same every time—there was no changing it, no swaying it to glorify any pieces of it or tie it up with a pretty pink bow. It was messy. It was real. It came pouring out of me the way anything real ever had before.

It was me, and now this eating disorder, and my transition from veganism—a diet and a lifestyle that had been a huge part of my life during a very definitive time in my brand-new semblance of adulthood—was now a part of me too. And holy hell, did it feel good to get it down on paper.

It was so special to write it down because I knew those words expressed my mindset and my struggles exactly as they were—no frills, no fillers to make it sound more interesting or easier to understand. If people disagreed with it, I would be fine because I would draw confidence from the fact that everything I said was straight from the heart. If anyone wanted to reject me because of it, I didn't want them reading my blog in the first place, and I certainly didn't want them in my life.

The next morning was a bit of a whirlwind. I had typed the post out on my computer, scheduled it to go live in the morning, and included photos along with the decorated "follow your heart" and "be yourself" quotes that had never held greater meaning to me than they did in that very moment. Right before I posted it, I had a phone conversation with a blogging friend of mine who has experienced great success with her vegan dessert blog. She supported my decision, and she talked me through what might happen when the post went live.

"You might get death threats," she warned. I was shocked and even a little flattered that she suggested people might care that much. I reminded myself that my blog wasn't anywhere near the level of hers, that even though I had a good number of readers, it wasn't on the massive scale she was used to. She also told me my site might crash because so much traffic would be directed to it, and again I made a mental note that no such thing seemed like it could happen with my blog.

We got off the phone, and even though she (among others) urged me to think long and hard about my decision to go public so soon, I needed to get the truth off my chest. So in true Jordan fashion, I hung up the phone with one hand and pressed the "Publish" button for the post with my other hand. I went straight to Instagram, where my seventy thousand followers were, and posted a photo with large block letters saying, "Why I'm Transitioning Away from Veganism . . . "

Public Reaction

What happened from there shocks me to this day. My website crashed immediately due to the heavy traffic from Instagram and the rapidly spreading word on the Internet. I spent two frantic hours on the phone, alternating between my hosting site and my web designer, all the while fielding angry comments on Instagram calling me a disgrace and a sell-out—before they could even *read* my explanation post! I felt naked, responding to these angry strangers with words that didn't do justice to what I had written the day before. When the site was finally back up, I breathed a major sigh of relief and directed them all there to get their explanation.

What I found when I got there was astonishing. My site had exceeded thirty-thousand views that morning alone, and it had only been back up for a matter of minutes. Comment after comment after comment expressed negativity, support, negativity, support, *extreme* negativity, *extreme* support, and everything in between. My email inbox was the same. It was filled with irate ethical vegans spewing hateful names at me and demanding their money back for cleanse programs they had bought from my site and T-shirts they had purchased from my clothing line, claiming they would never have supported a non-vegan vendor had they known the "*truth*."

And then there were the people I knew personally—people I went to high school or elementary school with, friends of friends of acquaintances of friends' relatives who were reaching out with touching stories of their own. I was blown away and moved to tears that people trusted me with their intensely personal stories and challenges related to food, eating disorders, exercise, and body image. Instantly I felt so much less alone. I went from having one friend who I was sure understood (plus plenty of amazing friends who understood as well as they could) to a whole cyberspace of supporters and comrades with whom to embark on this recovery journey.

But as great as the support was—and "great" is an understatement; it was over-the-moon mind-blowing and wonderful—the hatred still had to run its course. I had never experienced hateful comments in my life other than during the vegan honey controversy I had been through the year before. The extreme anger thrown my way by strangers and a large handful of people I thought were my friends was absolutely sickening.

I knew that when putting myself out there in such a public way, receiving criticism was par for the course. But the amount of disturbing negativity cast my way, almost 100 percent from the vegan community and the raw vegan community, was disheartening. In the beginning, it totally killed me. I couldn't believe I was losing readers and followers by the thousands, and that my own dietary choices could be responsible for legitimate death threats.

anger

"[MY INBOX] WAS FILLED WITH IRATE ETHICAL VEGANS SPEWING HATEFUL NAMES AT ME AND DEMANDING THEIR MONEY BACK FOR CLEANSE PROGRAMS THEY HAD BOUGHT FROM MY SITE AND T-SHIRTS THEY HAD PURCHASED FROM MY CLOTHING LINE, CLAIMING THEY WOULD NEVER HAVE SUPPORTED A NON-VEGAN VENDOR HAD THEY KNOWN THE '*TRUTH*.'"

It was particularly hard to accept because I had once been a part of that community and felt very embraced by it. I learned quickly that many of my vegan-centric friendships had been a façade based on dietary choices and went no deeper than our commonly shared label. I would never go so far as to say that "vegans" dislike me now because I know that there is *so much more* to a person than what they choose to eat and how they choose to live their life. I wish that people who let my dietary choices define my personality in their eyes would give me the same courtesy, but I understand now that sometimes people stretch the confines of a label to let it define much more than it actually does.

The cruel words launched my way from many in the vegan community were downright hateful. Lots of the people who lashed out were strangers, but good portions of them were also people I knew personally or had come to know through the vegan blogosphere. The comments ranged from death threats to belittling attacks about my weight, my family, and my character. Some people who were angry *tried* to keep an open mind by beginning their commentary by saying, "I truly believe you are a good person, *but . . .*" And for that I cannot fault them because they are so blinded by their dietary beliefs, they cannot see that someone's goodness is based on so much more than what they choose to eat.

I have had to learn to be very diplomatic in my responses to the people who write angry things to me. The first thing I learned was that responding is pretty unnecessary and is almost always a terrible idea—no matter what, the person will lash back with something even harsher than their original comment, and more than likely they will loop in some of their equally angry friends. I also learned that when I *do* respond, everything about my response will be picked apart. If I try to be understanding and kind, I'm criticized for being condescending. If I say screw it and stand up for myself, I'm told I'm acting overly emotional and defensive. In short, I'm damned if I do and damned if I don't.

Another thing I've learned is that there is no use reiterating the fact that veganism didn't cause my eating disorder because even though it's the truth and I've been putting it out there since the day I came public about my transition, people who are already angry don't want to hear it. They are upset that my story inevitably shone a negative light on veganism, and they want to blame my inner character for it. It's no fun for them to be upset *and* to have no one to blame.

I will preface this by saying I know many incredible vegans who have stood by me and supported my choices, but the truth must be told that in many cases, veganism can be an elitist way of thinking. I can't tell you how many times I've come across a vegan who likely despised me and who told me that eventually I would "come to my senses" and return to the diet. They're clearly unwilling to believe that perhaps I needed to let go of the restrictive way of life to regain my health and that my health is important. For me, veganism became restrictive. For many vegans, it never turns into a restrictive mentality. Isn't it worth mentioning that everyone is *different* and we should all find a way to eat and live that works best for us?

The group of vegans who dislike me and the balanced way of life I stand for will be the first to tell you that in their opinion, veganism isn't *about* feeling good, it's about preserving the lives of the innocent and being a voice for the voiceless. I would argue that veganism is different for everyone who is a part of it, just like being "healthy" or being a woman or being a musician is different for everyone who falls into each of those categories. Veganism, for me, was as much about feeling good as it was about anything else. If my reasoning doesn't fall into the traditional category of ethical veganism, I'm not going to apologize for it. I am not going to "take back" being a vegan just because some people claim that I never was because in their opinion you can't "stop" being vegan.

different

"I WOULD ARGUE THAT VEGANISM IS DIFFERENT FOR EVERYONE WHO IS A PART OF IT, JUST LIKE BEING 'HEALTHY' OR BEING A WOMAN OR BEING A MUSICIAN IS DIFFERENT FOR EVERYONE WHO FALLS INTO EACH OF THOSE CATEGORIES."

That closed-mindedness is what turns people off to veganism to begin with, which is okay with me even though it's too bad, but it is not okay with me that it also turns people away from living a healthy lifestyle. Even some of my highly educated friends and family who are less interested in health and fitness than I am still take quite a bit of convincing that sugar-free desserts can be delicious and that gluten-free pizza isn't as scary as it sounds. I know that part of the reason people associate certain healthy trends with extremism is because of the judgmental, holier-than-thou mentality that frequently comes along with them.

Well, let me tell you something. Being a gluten-free, sugar-free, oil-free, grain-free, legume-free, plant-based raw vegan didn't make me any better than anyone else. It made me restricted and emotionally exhausted, yes, and even if I *had* been getting enough nutrients to live that way forever, I never would have acted like I was better than anyone else who didn't eat that way. I think the only dietary style worth bragging about is eating in a way that makes you feel amazing, balanced, and healthy. Listening to your body is something to brag about. And if animal rights and environmental activism are two things you are passionate about on top of feeling good, don't let the extremists tell you that you can't make a positive change in those areas just because you don't eat a strictly vegan diet.

You can do whatever you want! Anyone who tells you otherwise is just a big bully, and I have a hunch that on top of being a bully they also have widespread insecurities of their own. People don't lash out when they are happy and confident in their own decisions. They just don't.

Coming Back

The first few days that I received the intense negativity, I was not only petrified, I was pretty much paralyzed with anxiety. I didn't sleep for three nights straight. I spent entire nights awake in my closet-size New York bedroom, my heart pounding so loud it was making me nauseous, on the phone with my web designer or my mom, depending on the hour, hysterically trying to decide on a new blog name and simultaneously trying not to panic about what breakfast would be the next morning.

Imagine beginning your eating-disorder recovery journey while people are calling you a "fat piece of lard" on a daily basis and telling you that you deserve to rot in hell along with your entire family. It leaves you no room to exist without inner strength, which became my blessing in disguise. Now, I like to thank my "haters" (who still very much like to hang around my site) for teaching me the art of deep reflection.

In one particular fit of panic in response to an onslaught of hateful comments from the high-carb, low-fat vegan community (a.k.a. the 80/10/10 diet of my short-lived experiment), I changed my blog name in the middle of the night from *The Blonde Vegan* to *The Blonde Veggie*.

I know, right? It makes basically no sense. I was trying to move away from labels, and I certainly wasn't trying to express that I was vegetarian, but in my exhaustion-diluted and panic-stricken mind, it was catchy. And it meant not having to let go of the TBV acronym I had grown to love and feel extremely attached to. I felt like it was unfair for that name, the name that defined the brand I had built, the first business venture of my own that was only beginning, to be taken away from me. Maybe it sounds dramatic now, but TBV was everything to me. A lot of other things were changing, and I was about to move back across the country, so letting go of the name TBV and everything it embodied felt all wrong.

Luckily, those who knew me well knew that *The Blonde Veggie* didn't exactly have the strong ring to it that my blog and growing business needed. I woke up the next morning to a few texts and calls from some close friends gently suggesting maybe I'd jumped the gun with that one. So name-wise it was back to the drawing board. I knew I wanted something that personified balance, but I also knew I didn't want to stray too far from the original name—so I basically had a couple of choices: *The Balanced Blonde*, *Balanced Blonde*, *Blonde and Balanced*, or *Balanced and Blonde*.

haters

"IMAGINE BEGINNING YOUR EATING-DISORDER RECOVERY JOURNEY WHILE PEOPLE ARE CALLING YOU A 'FAT PIECE OF LARD' ON A DAILY BASIS AND TELLING YOU THAT YOU DESERVE TO ROT IN HELL ALONG WITH YOUR ENTIRE FAMILY."

And I think you know which one I chose! The Balanced Blonde stood out from all those names as something I would feel proud to represent. It embodied the motto of balance that I was growing more and more infatuated with by the day. I knew I hadn't reached my own level of balance yet, but I was on the road, and writing about it and sharing it with others excited me.

So what did I do? I tracked down the lovely young girl who had the username "@thebalancedblonde" on Instagram (and by tracked her down, I mean I stalked the living daylights out of her by scrolling through her followers, finding her personal account, messaging her on Facebook, figuring out we had a mutual friend, and then getting her phone number to explain my entire situation), and when she kindly said I could have the name because she didn't use her account anymore, *The Balanced Blonde* was in action.

However, it took me months before I even reached that point. When I went on national television to discuss my transition a mere week after I came public about it on my blog, I was introduced by ABC's Juju Chang as "Jordan Younger, *The Blonde Veggie*." At first I was a little upset with myself that I chose a funny name in such haste that only ended up sticking for about a week or two, but now I look back and smile about all that the name encompasses. It was my fruitful attempt to take one step forward from veganism, but not too big of a step. It was my defensive response to the haters who called me a cowardly liar for holding on to the "vegan" part of my blog name for a few days longer than their liking, and it was my very Jordan-esque quick-fix answer to the deeper, more pressing question of *"What the hell do I do now???"*

I couldn't possibly have been prepared for the amount of attention that was given to the story, but I am endlessly grateful for it, and I completely understand where the intrigue comes from. I developed an eating disorder, orthorexia nervosa, that even my eating disorder therapist had hardly heard of and knew very little about. I silently self-diagnosed myself with the disorder after reading about it on the Internet, and that was months before my monumental eating disorder conversation with Tara. Orthorexia is not yet recognized by the *Diagnostic and Statistical Manual of Mental Disorders (DSM)* like more traditional eating disorders are, but I predict that with the rising health obsession in our modern lifestyle, it will only become more and more prevalent.

Orthorexia is the answer to what many of us believed to be was a personality-related anxiety issue surrounding food that could never truly be remedied. I for one thought I would live with it forever. The moment I broke the ties that bound me to a life of severe restriction, my world became instantly brighter. I had more options, vastly more, which became somewhat of an issue in itself for a while, but it's human to have options. To deny ourselves those options, especially when our body is begging for them, is blatantly wrong.

I believe that my story was also particularly intriguing to the media because there aren't a whole lot of long-term studies for the plant-based vegan diet. I am not here to offer my scientific advice to you about veganism because clearly that would be very out of place, but I am here to recount my own personal journey. After going through the ups and downs that led to a downturn in my physical and mental health, I can confidently say that veganism is not for me. It triggered a desire within me to be more and more extreme, more and more pure, and to achieve more and more nutritional *perfection* to the point where no foods were safe.

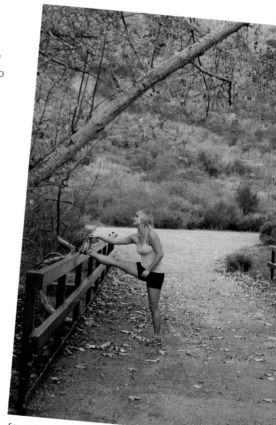

I understand that that is not what vegan-ism is to everyone. Some people can thrive on a vegan diet, even a plant-based vegan diet, and I find that typically those people do not harbor the same types of extreme personality traits that I do. I also find that thriving on a plant-based vegan diet takes a lot of hard work and dedi-cation, and some of us are not wired to devote that much time and effort to our food consumption. For some of us, it leaves no room for everything else in life—for relationships, for work, for exercise, for passions and hobbies such as writing and swimming and yoga and travel. Or maybe it does

SOMETIMES GETTING OUTSIDE AND MOVING ARE ALL I NEED TO GET MY THOUGHTS BACK ON TRACK.

leave room, but that space is tainted with an overarching anxiety of "Is there going to be anything for me to eat here, or am I just going to be screwed?"

For a period of time, I prided myself on being the type of person, the type of *plant-based vegan*, rather, that didn't care if there was anything for me to eat in any particular place. I would eat beforehand, I would bring my own food, or I wouldn't eat at all. It wasn't about the food, I told myself; it was about the people I was surrounding myself with.

But I later learned that when people are bonding over food and drinks and you exclude yourself from it, a sense of loneliness and isolation starts to creep up. You feel different, you feel like you can't fully join in, and try as they might, even your loved ones don't totally understand you. Maybe some people can deal with that! I thought I could for a long, long time. Far before I was vegan, even. I brought my own gluten-free snacks and treats on high school field trips and to dance competitions because I knew the rest of the food available wouldn't work for me. And that was fine—that was me listening to my body and knowing that the other food available would make me sick.

In my mid-twenties, I didn't want to keep avoiding food in general and avoiding restaurants and social gatherings with my friends because of unexplainable food anxieties and a strict dietary label I hardly agreed with anymore. It started to chip away at me a bit. It started to make me feel different in a way I didn't need. I was different enough as it was, being so extreme and having dietary restrictions to begin with; the last thing I needed to do was add fuel to the fire.

So I tried my best to move away from it. Coming forward was the first hurdle, and the support that came from that carried me over to my next hurdle.

12

WHAT'S GOING ON WITH ME?

A couple of months into my recovery process, I went through a brief period where I rejected healthy food in general. I don't mean I thought vegetables were the devil or I wouldn't let myself have a quinoa salad for lunch, but it was the in-betweens I obsessed about. I absolutely had to snack, or else I feared I would be starving come mealtime, and I still didn't know what that meant when chicken, fish, or even beef could be on the plate. If I was too hungry at dinner, what if I ate too much steak? Wouldn't that be *too much cholesterol*? I started snacking on foods I wouldn't have dreamed about while I was orthorexic so I could avoid those dreamed-up pitfalls.

During this period, for a few months over the summer when I moved back to California, I felt I absolutely had to try several foods per day that had previously been off-limits: ice cream, candy, even pizza and sandwiches and hamburgers (after all those years of avoiding gluten!). Every burger had to be followed by a frozen yogurt doused in toppings, which was becoming such a staple that my mom could sense my "We should go to fro-yo!" suggestion coming before it even came out of my mouth.

I bounced from the restrictive extreme to the other end of the spectrum: the stuff-myself-silly extreme. It actually makes me sick just thinking about it, not because I think any of the foods I tried and ate in abundance are "bad" or should be avoided in general, but because I was stuffing myself because I felt like I had no choice. I went from the vegan girl to the "recovering" girl overnight, and if I wasn't constantly testing myself and proving to myself and everyone around me that unhealthy food wasn't going to make me sick from the inside out, then I felt like I was doing something wrong or that I wasn't trying hard enough to get better.

If I posted a veggie-based meal on my Instagram or blog, I received an influx of comments ranging from "Hey, you're not vegan anymore . . . Why are you eating that?" to "I think you're going to become vegan again. Yay!!!" to "Maybe now she will finally lose some weight and be super skinny again." And yes, people actually refer to me as "she" on my own blog and social media accounts from time to time, which I find pretty annoying—I suppose there will always be Internet trolls of some sort.

That same summer, I traveled to Italy and the south of France with my family, and I couldn't have been more excited about the trip. I hadn't been to Europe since I had studied abroad in Florence in college, and I had spent the last two years wondering how hard it would be to ever travel in Europe again while navigating the eating situation. Now that I was opening myself to a whole new realm of foods, the idea of eating and enjoying the cultural aspect of food on the trip felt extra enticing and also nerve-wracking.

We went with a big group from my mom's side of the family, most of them very intrigued about what my diet now consisted of and what exactly I would eat on the trip. I started out moderately, just like my transition from veganism itself. I tried a few things here and a few things there: a slice of pizza in Sardinia, a gelato in Florence, a piece of chocolate cake on our cruise ship. I put on a brave face while I tried everything, but inside I was still suffering.

Since I was so open about my eating-disorder recovery experience, I felt like extra eyes were on me every time I ate. Even if it was in my head, it felt like others were always hyperaware of what I was going to put into my mouth. I couldn't order a dish or even peruse a menu without someone commenting about how different I must feel now that I'm not so restricted. If I finished the food on my plate, people noticed and remarked about it. If I only ate half, people wanted to know why. Did I not like it? Was it too far out of my comfort zone?

Europe was a real testing ground on that front. I was sharing a room with my mom and was with twenty family members from first thing in the morning to late at night, so there was really no hiding my still-strange eating habits. My mom has always been great at being aware of my food issues without casting her own judgment or opinions and also without making a big deal about them; she knows that is not effective with me. (By the way, I don't think making a big deal out of anyone's food issues is very effective!)

On this trip in particular, my mom knew I was in the early stages of recovery, which meant there was a lot of panic and discomfort surrounding food. Just like I did when I was in the throes of my eating disorder, I packed a month's supply of protein bars and processed-free snacks in my suitcase "just in case" the food I was comfortable eating wouldn't be readily available. The problem was, I was in a quandary about whether to eat said protein bars or just go with the flow and eat the Italian and French cuisine for every meal without stressing.

I was so used to eating differently than everyone else. Learning that maybe I didn't *need* those protein bars and that I no longer had to keep an apple in my purse or save it for a starvation emergency was hard. And beyond that, it was uncomfortable. I was so, so accustomed to obsessing about food. The obsession was an outlet for my nervous energy and my deeper food issues.

In Italy and France, it also became clear that while several of my food obsessions still remained, they didn't always make a whole lot of sense. For instance, I was panic-stricken about trying pasta or anything too carb-heavy on the trip, but I was pretty comfortable with eating dessert every night and going back for seconds at the breakfast buffet. I didn't feel *great* about having so much dessert when all things refined sugar had been so strictly off-limits for years, but the fact that I was eating it at all was noticeable to me in comparison with the pasta.

hyperaware

"SINCE I WAS SO OPEN ABOUT MY EATING-DISORDER RECOVERY EXPERIENCE, I FELT LIKE EXTRA EYES WERE ON ME EVERY TIME I ATE. EVEN IF IT WAS IN MY HEAD, IT FELT LIKE OTHERS WERE ALWAYS HYPERAWARE OF WHAT I WAS GOING TO PUT INTO MY MOUTH."

I knew it made no sense to everyone around me that pasta equaled gluttony in my mind, but chocolate cake was acceptable. To understand my own logic, I had to dig deep to find the root of the problem. I knew that part of the reason I avoided pasta was because gluten never made me feel good, and I knew better than to test those boundaries and then feel sick later. I also had not-so-great memories of eating ravioli, spaghetti, and gnocchi in overabundance when I studied abroad in Florence. It seemed, when I look back on studying abroad in college, that I was controlling my anxiety even back then through food—and I then began to associate that reliance and extreme mentality with pasta in general. This was the beginning of me starting to listen to my body—avoiding gluten not because it wasn't *allowed*, but because it didn't make me feel good.

So, needless to say, although I was making strides with trying new foods, I was still stuck in my head and trying to figure out my relationship with food in my newfound label-free life. It frustrated me that I still felt so *off* when I was listening to my body by eating more protein and foods rich in the B_{12} vitamins I was deficient in. When I looked in the mirror, I saw a bloated, scared, and overwhelmed version of myself that didn't at all match up with who I wanted to be or who I was used to being. I felt like I had no idea what to eat and what not to eat—the wide-open world of food was too much to handle when I was so used to being in my plant-based vegan box.

Now I was at a new crossroads. I was proud that I enjoyed the Italian and French food and culture as much as my recovering body would allow, but I also felt lost on a new level. *Why* was I eating in a seemingly balanced way and still feeling like crap? What was I doing wrong? I wanted to get back to a place where I had more energy and didn't feel like I had five or ten pounds (2.3 to 4.5 kg) of excess "confusion weight" hanging on. I knew it was better than the alternative, the painful obsessions and starvation, but I also knew I was still suffering from orthorexia and it had just taken on a different form—a form in which I was forcing myself to try new things, yet was continuously disappointed with what felt like a lack of discipline.

Also on that trip, I was still dealing with the backlash from my dietary switch. I had recently appeared on *Good Morning America*, *Nightline*, and *NPR* and in *Teen Vogue*, *People*, *ELLE Australia*, and similar outlets discussing my transition; ethical vegans were not happy. Between the angry emails and the contrasting wonderful outpouring of support from fellow sufferers and people who recognized themselves or their loved ones in my story, my inbox was out of control. Email was a huge part of my business, the way I secured any partnerships for my blog, and now that even my inbox was an overflowing mess, I felt like I was drowning.

I needed help, and I needed it quick. I just didn't know what help looked like, just as I didn't know what reaching my health goals was going to look like. I pretty much knew one thing and one thing only: I wanted to share this story with as many people as possible. I wanted to show people who suffer from eating disorders, especially orthorexia and any type of EDNOS (eating disorder not otherwise specified), that they are not alone—that there is a way out. I knew that the first step was rejecting my dietary label in favor of listening to my body. I had talked to countless readers from around the world, thousands at this point, who had developed a form of orthorexia due to a labeled diet of some sort.

I did my best to spread the word that strict dietary regimens, even if they are deemed "the healthiest way to live" by various studies and doctors and opinionated individuals, should be avoided by anyone with as extreme of a personality as my own. So many of us should stay far away from self-inflicted extremes in an already-challenging world, and I felt there was a gap where people should be discussing what an issue dietary theories had become. If you search "healthy diet" on the Internet, you'll be met with an onslaught of contradictory information. Some people will tell you to eat as the cavemen once did while others will scoff and say we are far more evolved and should eat only plants. And, of course, there is everything else in between and then some.

challenge

"SO MANY OF US SHOULD STAY FAR AWAY FROM SELF-INFLICTED EXTREMES IN AN ALREADY-CHALLENGING WORLD, AND I FELT THERE WAS A GAP WHERE PEOPLE SHOULD BE DISCUSSING WHAT AN ISSUE DIETARY THEORIES HAD BECOME."

I felt desperate to let people know that by trying to be as healthy as they can be in an *extreme* way, which clearly seems like a good idea to anyone up for the challenge, maybe they were actually damaging their health in the long run. I knew I still needed to find my own answers, but spreading the message of balance helped me see my own recovery with more clarity.

I researched all my options. I continued seeing doctor after doctor, nutritionist after nutritionist, and then acupuncturists, colonic hydrotherapists, wellness coaches, holistic healers, and gastroenterologists. I knew that letting go of the intense restriction of plant-based veganism was a good first step, but I didn't know what was going to be next. I felt like I'd tried everything, and going on another strict diet of any kind was out of the question. Labels confined me, and if I was clear on one thing, it was that they no longer had any suitable place in my life.

Then, amid all the confusion, I got sick—this time in a way that clearly had to do with the food I had been putting into my body. After years of restriction and the deficiencies I'd developed, my body stopped producing the enzymes necessary to digest foods such as dairy, meat, and poultry. It wasn't something I noticed at first because I truly did feel great when I started eating some of those previously off-limits foods again for the first time, but over the course of several months, my stomach started feeling off—way off.

In the beginning, I thought I was coming down with the flu. It was October, and I had been off my vegan diet for about five months. I had just started eating red meat again about once a week and had been eating fish, poultry,

restriction

"AFTER YEARS OF RESTRICTION AND THE DEFICIENCIES I'D DEVELOPED, MY BODY STOPPED PRODUCING THE ENZYMES NECESSARY TO DIGEST FOODS SUCH AS DAIRY, MEAT, AND POULTRY."

and yogurt pretty consistently. I tried to push forward in my recovery and keep my mindset open, but I was in a lot of physical pain. The bottom of my stomach was filled with a hollow, nauseated, bloated feeling. The sensation vacillated between standard discomfort and feeling like it was on fire. Then the pain worked its way up to my chest as well, and now there were two fires—one in my stomach and one right over my heart.

I complained about it relentlessly. I was home in Sacramento for a few weeks in early October, so it was my parents who had to listen to the brunt of it. The pain was exhausting, and even though I was supposed to drive back to LA to resume my regular life and leap back into the health and wellness blogosphere, I hardly had enough energy to move from my bed to the couch. I decided to extend my stay at home indefinitely—at least until I could figure out what was wrong.

I was used to having stomach pain. It went away for several months in the beginning of my plant-based transition, but even when I was eating in that clean, vegan manner, the stomach problems cropped back up. I was also used to the people around me not understanding, which I didn't blame them for, but it still frustrated me. I felt I had to assert my pain extra loudly and clearly in order for my parents to take me seriously, so one morning in particular I woke up with my mind set to do just that.

"I still feel really sick," I said to my mom, who was surprisingly already in the hallway on the way to my room when I woke up. And then, for emphasis, I added, "I'm *very* concerned."

"I am too," she said. "I think I finally know what's wrong."

She went on to explain that she had been researching my symptoms the night before, and every single one of them could be explained by stomach ulcers. My immediate reaction was panic (including a minor fainting episode), but my second reaction was immense relief. If she was right, it would mean I could go on medication and get better. Maybe that explained the major imbalance I had been feeling, and if I was extra lucky, maybe it even explained a childhood of stomach problems and imbalance as well.

We tried to get in with my doctor immediately, but because he didn't have any appointments that day, we settled for seeing a physician's assistant. I was very used to the routine of going to the doctor, explaining to the physician, the nurse, the PA, whoever was there to listen, what I was pretty damn sure I had. I'd had enough stomach issues over the years to gain a pretty decent grasp on what was causing my pain and what wasn't, and this ulcer business sounded very legitimate.

The PA agreed that we were probably right about the ulcers, so he put me on a trial run of acid-blocking medication (a proton pump inhibitor) and a medley of other pills to coat my stomach four times a day before eating. I downed the drugs immediately, and for a few days I started feeling a little better. At this point, I was also extremely routine about what I could and could not eat—acidic foods were a no-no—and that seemed to be helping too.

I was trying my best not to get fanatical about this new diet regimen. I was still in the middle of my recovery process, and a big part of me knew I needed to ditch the restrictions and just *live*. For a few weeks, I ate in this very careful, acid-free way, tentatively, paralyzed by the fear of the returning ulcer pain. My TBB iPhone app was about to come out, which meant the culmination and celebration of lots of hard work for my app developer and me.

By the time our launch party came around, I was feeling a bit better. I had been subsisting on eggs, cottage cheese, avocado, chicken, and oatmeal for a good three weeks, and the routine had me feeling pretty darn proud of myself. I knew I had lost a few pounds (1 to 2 kg), and even though I still had a dull pain in my lower stomach, I felt like I was on the right track.

But, as all restrictive tendencies do, this one was wearing thin, and I could feel the weight of it. Planning the party was a massive responsibility, and when the day came around, I lost the time to eat lunch, and then I lost the

fanatical

"I WAS TRYING MY BEST NOT TO GET FANATICAL ABOUT THIS NEW DIET REGIMEN. I WAS STILL IN THE MIDDLE OF MY RECOVERY PROCESS, AND A BIG PART OF ME KNEW I NEEDED TO DITCH THE RESTRICTIONS AND JUST *LIVE*."

time to eat dinner. The party itself was wonderful, and I was blown away by the number of people who came out to support. Once the night ended, I was on an adrenaline high, and even though I hadn't eaten since breakfast, when my app developer suggested we get a late bite somewhere, I felt my stomach sink. No way. It can't happen this late at night, I thought, not after so much excitement and so many hours of stomach emptiness.

Plus, I realized that the whole ulcer thing had become a handy excuse for why I couldn't eat normally, why I couldn't drink alcohol, and why my life still had to kind of, sort of revolve around food no matter what. But instead of dragging on like this for two years like I did with veganism, I barely lasted one month on my "ulcer diet."

When it became clear that the medication didn't do its job, my doctors and I realized that a stomach ulcer couldn't be the culprit. I went back to the gastroenterologist, this time learning about small intestinal bacterial overgrowth (SIBO), a condition in which abnormally large amounts of bacteria are present in the small intestine. SIBO causes all the symptoms I had previously attributed to stomach ulcers, including abdominal pain, bloating, feeling "off balance," and digestive and absorption issues.

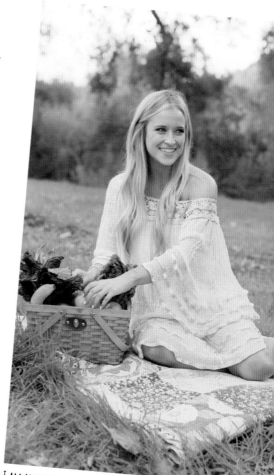

I AM ALWAYS THE GIRL WHO BRINGS HEALTHY FOOD TO A PICNIC OR PARTY—THAT WON'T CHANGE.

Soon thereafter I took a SIBO breath test and learned I did in fact have bacteria in my small intestine that didn't belong there. On top of that, my stomach was lacking in certain important digestive enzymes from my restrictive dietary days. The food I had been eating, stuffing my face with, rather, throughout the middle of my recovery was too much for my damaged system to handle. A two-week dose of SIBO antibiotics, and more importantly, a heavy round of digestive enzymes started working together to get my stomach back on track. It didn't make a huge difference in the way I felt, but it was enough to help me reflect on what worked and what didn't work for me and to rededicate myself to being healthy without being obsessive.

Now I finally had the tools I needed to listen to my body. Without my stomach rebelling against everything I ate, I was able to move forward and find balance in a new way: a way that was not rooted in food obsessions, lifelong intolerances, stomach sensitivities, or reactive conditions. I could just be. Or at least I could try, in my own extreme way, to begin feeling what it might be like to *just be me*.

13

REAL SUGAR, WHAT?!

While I was recovering, I cut way back on time in the kitchen. In the height of my orthorexic days, everything in my world revolved around cooking, baking, recipe developing, food photography, food writing, and planning far in advance what I was going to actually *eat* versus what I was just going to make for the blog. And if I wasn't focused on all that, I was focusing on how I was going to burn off anything I'd just eaten.

Stepping away from my obsession to create in the kitchen was helpful in the beginning stages of my recovery, but part of me missed cooking and food photography as a creative outlet. My readers frequently mentioned how much they missed the recipes on my blog, and my friends not so subtly hinted that they wouldn't mind having my healthy baked goods lying around my apartment like they used to.

The reason the decrease was so noticeable is because I didn't just cut back on recipe developing and recipe blog posts; I avoided them entirely. I wrote just one recipe post in a five-month period, after consistently posting recipes five days a week for nearly a year. Once I was far enough into my recovery to recognize that I could cook and bake again without the fear of having excess food around, I decided it was time to experiment with something new.

I was pretty comfortable making smoothies, acai bowls, raw desserts, and veggie dishes for the blog, because even during the early stages of my recovery, I was hard at work creating plant-based dishes for the app I had already agreed to do before I transitioned my diet. Something I wasn't at all comfortable with, aside from attempting to make chicken and fish dishes (I still struggle with those!), was *refined sugar*.

Sugar Spotlight

I should add that refined sugar is nothing to idealize. Some people suffer from sugar addiction, and eating a diet high in sugar means having an excess of empty calories in our diet. But on the flip side, for someone recovering from an eating disorder and trying to reverse an all-out *fear* of refined sugar, demystifying it and showing yourself that you can have whatever you want in moderation is *much* healthier and more freeing for your mind (and body!) in the long run.

Even writing it now triggers those sinful, off-limits feelings I used to get so strongly whenever I thought about any form of sugar that wasn't derived from stevia, honey, agave syrup, coconut nectar, or *maybe*, if I was feeling wild, date sugar. After being in recovery for about six months, I was finally getting comfortable eating foods with refined sugars, like frozen yogurt and the occasional baked good, but my issue was with making them myself and actually witnessing the sugar going into them. Without knowing the details, at least I could kind of pretend.

I had always idolized bloggers who seemed to have no fear of the sugar content in their recipes. Yeah, I felt that some of the combos of butter, sugar, flour, and oil they used were kind of outdated and could be replaced with healthier alternatives, but that didn't take away the deep-rooted and silent jealousy I felt when I perused their websites and imagined them indulging in their decadent desserts with no anxiety or hesitation. And for all I knew, some of them might not have even touched their desserts after they made them and photographed them, but in my mind I felt that if they were making it, they had to be more comfortable around it than I would have been.

It took me *months* of back-and-forth deliberation before I finally decided to create a recipe with brown sugar in it. Before that, every time I got close I became overwhelmed with the fear of having too much of the potential dessert in my apartment and subsequently talked myself out of it. I would have intense flashbacks to the difficult orthorexic days when I created raw vegan desserts and ate every single bite of them after photographing them—usually because I was *starving* and was halfway shocked that I was allowing myself to eat solid food at all!

I knew it would be healthier to create a sugary dessert at home than to order one at a bakery or a restaurant, but I also knew that watching myself pour in the brown sugar the recipe called for might trigger something very anxious and fearful inside me. Regardless, I decided it was time, and I knew when I was finally ready. I needed to ease my mind a bit and show myself that if I could eat a cup (245 g) of frozen yogurt with toppings from a yogurt place down the street, then I could bake a batch of chocolate chip cookies and enjoy them just as much.

Plus, I needed to show myself I could enjoy them without eating the whole entire batch out of pure anxiety and the desire to get them out of my kitchen. And it was exciting to think about making and photographing something I knew my readers would enjoy. I had really missed the cooking aspect of blogging, and I knew I had it in me to bring my readers something *balanced* but decadent at the same time.

What I decided to do was put my own spin on a gluten-free chocolate chip cookie recipe. It included brown sugar—the *real* kind, and organic and fair trade to boot—and real chocolate chips (not dairy-free! Gasp!), but I substituted the white flour with almond flour and the canola oil with coconut oil,

balanced

"I HAD REALLY MISSED THE COOKING ASPECT OF BLOGGING, AND I KNEW I HAD IT IN ME TO BRING MY READERS SOMETHING *BALANCED* BUT DECADENT AT THE SAME TIME."

and I added in a few big scoops of almond butter to up the protein content. I couldn't entirely get rid of my desire to make healthier alternatives! There's a big difference between orthorexia and a passion for health.

Becoming My Own Best Friend

As I was mixing everything together, I vacillated between telling myself "See, you can make something delicious and satisfying while also keeping some of the nutritional value! You go, girl!" and "Holy *crap*, these aren't going to be very healthy, so I need to be really careful about how much of them I eat." Similarly, I was going back and forth between bursting with pride for making something so out of my comfort zone and bubbling with concern for what the heck would happen once these cookies were actually baked and cooling on the counter, staring me in the face, no doubt.

I tried as much as I could to put the anxious thoughts out of my mind so I could attempt to enjoy the experience and let it be as cathartic as possible. It was my first time baking anything with sugar in *years*, so I knew what I really needed to focus on was being kind to myself and nonjudgmental about whatever was to come from it. It would be a learning experience, and no matter what happened, I would come out of it with a greater awareness of myself and where I was in my recovery process.

After combining all the ingredients and tasting the dough, one of my first thoughts was *whoa*, real cookie dough tastes a hell of a lot better than the "cookies" I'd been throwing together for the past few years with oats, almond butter, mashed banana, and cacao nibs. My second thought was . . . *This* is what I have been so worried about?! This is a cakewalk!

It was a really cool feeling to soak in that wave of realization. Food is food. Food fuels us, we should enjoy it, and we should not let it get in the way of our lives. For a food blogger, it has a lot more complication to it, as our jobs are pulled into it too, but at the end of the day, it is something we need and something we should have a good relationship with. It took this cookie-dough-tasting experience for me to add yet another missing piece of recovery awareness to my ever-growing puzzle.

The baking itself didn't go quite as smoothly as the batter tasting. I wasn't entirely sure how long to leave the cookies in the oven, since it had been a long, long time since I had baked anything with real eggs in it, and once

Puzzle Talk

Speaking of puzzles, all this talk about adding pieces of awareness to my recovery puzzle reminds me of when I was in third grade and I was home sick with pneumonia and whooping cough for three months. My mom sat on my floor day in and day out, working on a huge, twenty-thousand-piece puzzle that was a re-creation of a painting of little girl in the forest. She worked on that damn puzzle every minute of every day because she was so afraid to leave my room (I was really sick!), but she didn't want to scare me by hovering over me. Her diligence when I was sick and her unwavering dedication to making sure I got better was something I drew upon as strength when I was recovering from my eating disorder more than fifteen years later. It's crazy how much we remember the strength shown to us in the dark times. I have no doubt that her support this time around will be equally memorable fifteen years from now and beyond.

they started expanding and getting golden brown along the edges, I decided it was time to take them out. Really what I was experiencing was a major panic about leaving them in for too long, and I was having some anticipation issues because of my mental hype around the situation.

I wasn't super concerned about how they were going to turn out aesthetically because I already knew my plan was to crumble them and put them into a jar for a "Half-Baked Gluten-Free Cookies in a Jar" recipe post, but I was pretty concerned about how they were going to taste. The anxiety that started to take over my insides while they were baking prompted me to take them out far too soon and also to begin tasting them before they were even partially cooled. The cookies were totally stuck to the aluminum foil they'd been baking on top of, and I was so eager to get them into their jars I just accepted the huge mess that took place while I frantically scraped them.

However, even though the final product was a bit of a mess for me psychologically, it didn't entirely matter, because my *reaction* to the mess had changed. I was sort of upset that I hadn't been able to let the first batch finish cooking, and I was also sort of upset that I ate a *few* too many of them when they were straight out of the oven (okay, upwards of half a batch). But I didn't get extremely down on myself about it, and I certainly didn't judge my choices at all.

I totally understood why the situation was so difficult to deal with. I knew before I decided to make the cookies that it was going to be a struggle, and that's why I wanted to do it. I wanted to face the challenge, and I especially wanted to do it so I could get over the hump and start feeling a little more normal about sugar in general. I was kind to myself, and I reacted the way I would to a friend who was recovering from an eating disorder. I would never tell that friend they'd done anything wrong by getting anxious in the situation. I would praise them for challenging themselves and remind them how much easier it will get with time.

So that's exactly what I did with myself. I was finally able to begin practicing the art of being my own best friend. And that was much more valuable than my previous tactic of avoiding sugar at all costs.

The other thing was, even though I felt bad that I overindulged right off the bat, I had a much more normal reaction to the second and third batches, and I photographed them both inside and outside for well over an hour without the anxiety of feeling like I needed to try more. I let myself have my fix,

normalcy

"I WANTED TO FACE THE CHALLENGE, AND I ESPECIALLY WANTED TO DO IT SO I COULD GET OVER THE HUMP AND START FEELING A LITTLE MORE NORMAL ABOUT SUGAR IN GENERAL."

and then I was done. When I made vegan pumpkin chocolate chip "cookie dough" in New York nearly a year before, I panicked after overindulging and forced myself to eat more and then throw the rest away (a whole batch worth!) so I didn't need to deal with having it in my apartment anymore.

This is what I learned from the experience: I think it's very normal to eat cookie dough when you bake, and I would even take it a step further and say I think you *should*! I once read on the blog of someone who had suffered from an eating disorder in the past that she now eats too much cookie dough whenever she bakes and is proud of it because doing so would have sent her into a tailspin when she was sick. I read her article when I was in the middle of my eating disorder, and I was horrified. *Proud* of eating too much cookie dough? I could hardly imagine such a thing. I was torn between judging her for being unhealthy and envying everything about her approach.

But hey, now I get it. Maybe my cookie dough eating means I'm finally getting a little more normal. And if I had overindulged in cookie dough in the past, I certainly would have planned to skip dinner or at least have a juice or a protein shake in place of solid food later on. But I ate a full dinner that night, and I felt great. I did it because I was hungry, and I wanted it, and I knew it's what my body needed.

Imagine that.

14

LIVING WITH MY EXTREMES & MOVING FORWARD

What I've Learned:

- Self-hatred is an ugly thing. It should be replaced with forgiveness and self-respect.

- I need to surround myself only with good people who make me better every day.

- I am an emotional person by nature and need to take time to myself to unwind.

- I will continue to let go of my attachment to my eating disorder and the extreme mentality that came along with it . . . and that is the best and only thing I can do.

There is a lot more to say. This is not the end of my journey, but I am comfortable ending it here because there will never be an end. I will evolve and I will grow with the ebb and flow of what I learn and the new pieces of awareness I absorb along the way. I am changed because now I am open to soaking in what I learn about myself and my body without judgment, and I am aware of my thoughts and my feelings surrounding my health in a whole new way. I will never again shut myself off from understanding that I am suffering, either physically or emotionally, and I will not let my mind-body connection disappear as it once did. Instead I will work to strengthen it, and I will make an effort to be kind to myself every single day—even if it means forfeiting a green juice for a warm, gooey frosted cupcake or vice versa, depending on the day.

Learning to *listen* to my body has been key in my recovery process. It's not easy, but prioritizing that seemingly simple little fact is extremely valuable and worthwhile. Sometimes my body's signals are hard to understand, especially because in the months and years after an eating disorder a whole lot of junk can be out of whack. I had to work on getting my digestive enzymes restored, my hormones back in check, my blood sugar stabilized, and my hunger cues intact before I could even think about *really* listening to my body.

It's no freaking wonder that being aware of what my body wanted was so hard at the end of my vegan journey! And learning to listen is a journey in itself. But instead of taking it as a sprint (which, come on, let's be real, was *obviously* my first instinct), I have slowly but surely accepted that learning to listen to my body should be treated like a marathon: one step after the other, after the other, after the other. And when I get tripped up, instead of turning back and forcing myself to start from square one, I try to be kind to myself. I take a little break, almost like a breather, and then I hop back into the race. It's taken years of trial and error, but viewing it as a self-discovery challenge instead of the painstaking journey I once believed it to be has made a world of difference.

In a discussion I had a few months back with Dr. Steven Bratman, who coined the term *orthorexia* and subsequently, little did he know it, paved the way for my life to change, he told me something I have very much held on to. In his own recovery from orthorexia, he made a rule for himself that he wasn't allowed to spend more than 25 percent of his time thinking about food. When he first told me that, the percentage seemed impossible. How on earth could I bring something down from taking up 100 percent of the space in my mind to a mere fourth of that?

prioritize

"LEARNING TO *LISTEN* TO MY BODY HAS BEEN KEY IN MY RECOVERY PROCESS. IT'S NOT EASY, BUT PRIORITIZING THAT SEEMINGLY SIMPLE LITTLE FACT IS EXTREMELY VALUABLE AND WORTHWHILE."

But I tried, using him and his strength as my inspiration, and it's something I continue to try and carry out every single day. I know life is too precious to waste time panicking about what my next meal is going to look like, what the caloric content of a smoothie is down to the decimal, and how that might affect my health down the line. Life is meant to be enjoyed, squeezed, *balanced*, treasured, and magically different day after day. It's not meant to be predicted or rigid or dull—at least not the kind of life I want to live.

And life, life is going to be painful at times. It's going to be hard, and we are going to feel different and alone and entirely in over our heads. It's during those times that we need to trust ourselves most, to love ourselves, and to draw from previous experiences where we have brought our heads above water and done the damn thing no matter how hard it was. The quiet moments, the ones at the end of each day, when everyone else is gone or asleep or doing their own thing, that's when the magic happens. When we are forced to be strong or to break. And it's okay to break—it's only in breaking that we learn to pick ourselves back up again. And I'm beginning to see that it gets easier and easier each time, even if the struggles remain the same.

I don't know about you, but I would much rather enjoy a whopping slice of my niece's oozing chocolaty birthday cake, eat too much of it, and laugh with her about the frosting turning our teeth blue, than pace the side of the table, fifteen pounds (6.8 kg) lighter, and be *that* aunt

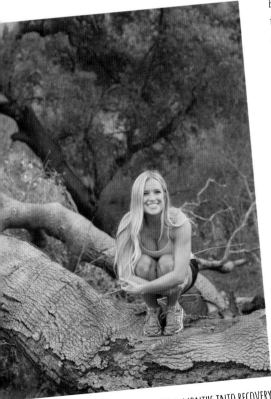

THIS SMILE IS REAL, SEVERAL MONTHS INTO RECOVERY.

(and friend and sister and daughter, while I'm at it) who just can't seem to live in the moment. And deep down, I was always that carefree being at my core, and I think that's a big reason why I was so motivated to climb back out of my sickness. I needed to be me again.

Just because I've recovered from the worst of my eating disorder doesn't mean I've magically transformed into an entirely balanced version of myself overnight. I will always have a bit of extremeness to my name, and that's not something I'm unhappy about. It means I love deeply and fight hard for what I believe in. Sure, sometimes it means that I am a panicked mess in the middle of the night or that I get so excited I forget to sleep, but that cavernous sensitivity and deep passion for what I do and who I surround myself with is part of what makes me who I am. Instead of changing it, I am learning to live with it.

I am learning to find *balance*, even if I have to dig it out from my totally extreme core. And call me crazy, but the road itself, now that I am out of the thick of it, has been kind of fun. It's a challenge, and I would take a challenge, no matter how unpredictable my day to day might be, over my militant and restrictive former lifestyle any day.

So for all of us who have ever found ourselves stuck, sick, labeled, extreme, afraid (okay, fine, terrified), and totally confused about what our next move is going to be—know that it's all going to be okay. There is no magic pill, but that's the best thing about it. Realizing that we are all so different and that there is no cure-all or one-size-fits-all answer to our deepest, darkest questions and fears, that's where we will start to grow. All it takes is a little bit of soul searching, a willingness to evolve, and a whole lot of compassion. Oh, and let's not forget . . . a healthy dose of balance doesn't hurt.

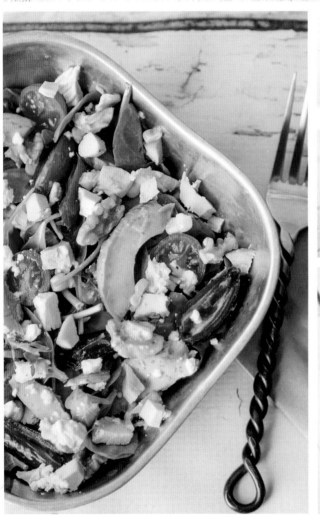
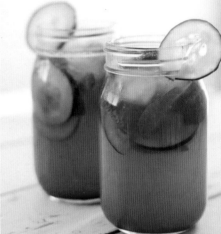
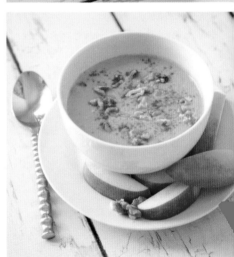

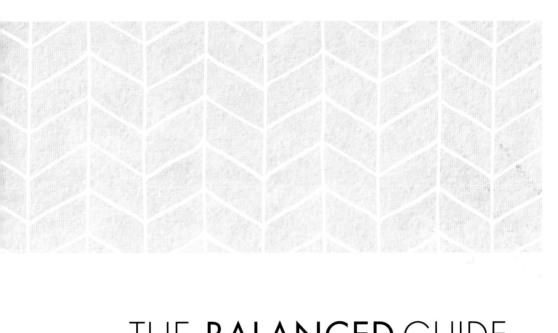

THE **BALANCED** GUIDE

PART 2

Living & Eating Well

Now Here Comes the Fun Stuff!

I gave you all the dirty details on how veganism triggered a serious eating disorder for me and how I lost my balance in the process. As a Libra, a person who constantly strives to find and maintain balance, striking it in my life after a long, rocky road of imbalance feels like coming home. It has taken a lot of work, but I prioritize the balance of food, exercise, relationships, and my overall lifestyle and happiness and check in with myself about it every single day. I am certainly not perfect, but the thing is . . . I'm not trying to be—and I don't think you should either.

I am simply trying to be the happiest, healthiest version of myself. And contrary to what I believed for many years, being the healthiest version of myself does *not* mean I am eating the cleanest diet under the sun. It means I am listening to my body, indulging in my cravings, and allowing myself to let loose and have wild nights out with friends (yes, nights that include alcohol) without beating myself up the next day or being so riddled with guilt, I can't even concentrate on anything else.

Balance sometimes means forgoing a cupcake in favor of a green juice, and other times it means saying no to a green juice because you want the damn cupcake. It means finding the rhythm within your own body to know what is going to serve you best in that moment, day, week, or month. For instance, when I am extra anxious, I tend to lose my appetite. Instead of forcing food down my throat where it will inevitably be met with acid and tummy problems (because my I carry all my anxiety in my stomach, like many of us do), I try to be gentle and drink lots of liquids and warm water with lemon; I also have light lunches and dinners.

On the flip side, I have had to learn through extreme trial and error not to use my anxious stomach as an excuse to deprive myself. For so many years, I lost my appetite due to anxiety and allowed it to spiral me into a borderline-anorexic, restrictive, food-obsessed zombie. And this restriction has never led me to anything other than hunger, brain fog, weakness, fatigue . . . and eventually stuffing my face with the nearest meal I could get my hands on, whether it was going to feel good on my stomach or not.

Maintaining balance relies on finding balance in the first place. If you're anything like me, finding that initial balance is the hardest part of the journey. Once you're on a good path, though, you will totally get on a roll. One balanced meal leads to the next, which leads to the next, and, what do ya know, even the next. When you're fueling yourself with balanced meals, you will have more energy to stay active and do the types of exercise you love. You will have more confidence and vitality to be present in your relationships and your work life and to learn new things. All in all, eating a balanced diet is part of the puzzle but, as opposed to what I once believed, it is not the *root* of all happiness—it is a piece. An important piece . . . just like the rest of the awesome components that make up your life.

In this section, I have provided you with a guide to what I believe are the most important steps toward finding and maintaining balance. There are balanced lifestyle tips, balanced recipes, and a handy little wrap-up to condense the tips into one solid, overarching message. Come back to these pages when you feel like you have deprived yourself for too long and need some help to get back on track or when you just need some extra motivation for eating whole, nourishing foods.

Please note that this isn't a weight loss guide or a "twenty-five recipes to change your life in twenty-five days" kind of deal. It's a lifestyle guide, and it's meant to provide you with the foundations to lead a happier, more confident, and entirely sustainable life when it comes to food, exercise, and learning to live life in moderation.

I'm no expert, and I am certainly not taking the place of your doctor, but on top of my health coaching certification, I am someone who has very much walked in the shoes of imbalance, and I know what it's like to feel completely and utterly helpless when it comes to making food choices. I have been on the extreme ends of the spectrum, I have been to raw vegan food restriction hell and back, and I know that for me, and my fellow extreme peeps, moderation is the way to go.

Balance. Let's find it. Let's maintain it. Let's kick our disordered eating habits' butts! Ready? It's time.

15

THE BALANCED LIFESTYLE GUIDE

A tried-and-true lesson I have learned throughout this whole process is that exercising balance in one area of your life and neglecting it in others will *not* lead you toward an overarching life of balance. If you tend to push things to the extreme, you may trick yourself into thinking that balance in one part of your life only (whether it be diet, exercise, or something else) will lead you directly down the path to ultimate health and happiness. Wouldn't that be nice?

Setting goals for health, wellness, and fitness certainly helps, but those are only small pieces of a larger whole. Achieving balance is just as much in the lifestyle as it is in the food and workout categories of our lives. If you're anything like me and you've gotten caught in one extreme or another, you might see the word *lifestyle* and think to yourself, "What in the world does that even *mean*? What falls under the umbrella of a healthy, balanced lifestyle other than food and fitness?"

Well, quite a few things. Relationships? Yep. Work-life balance? You bet. Hobbies? Mmm-hmm. Wait, even pursuing our passions, facing our fears, exploring new places, and experiencing new things? That's right, everything!

You might eat the most balanced diet in the whole entire universe (whatever that phrase means to you), but is the rest of your life getting the attention it deserves too? Do you have people to enjoy your health with? Do you treat yourself to things you love? Do you connect with yourself on a spiritual level, maybe in a way that makes you smile when you're alone in the car jamming out to your fave tunes? Speaking of that, are you okay with being alone?

Just to make sure you are on the right track when it comes to finding that balanced lifestyle we all crave and deserve, I have put together a sweet little Balanced Lifestyle Guide you can reference when you're feeling a little lost (or just need some inspiration).

You've got this. I promise.

Balanced Lifestyle Principles

The list starts with the most important, core lifestyle principles, so go in order if you can. When you've had your fill, take a walk and think about how you can incorporate these elements into your life before reading on.

BE YOUR OWN BEST FRIEND

Seriously, be comfortable with yourself! Have you ever heard the expression "What you eat in private, you wear in public"? Well also, what you *do* in private, you embody in public. If you sit around getting down on yourself and second-guessing your every move, you will emanate negativity and low self-confidence. On the other hand, if you wake up, tell yourself you're beautiful, and down a gingery green juice like you mean it, you will radiate the same confidence in public.

Living in New York taught me wonders about learning not only to be comfortable with myself, but also to enjoy my own company in the quiet moments. If you can *trust* your own opinions and reactions, you have a lifelong confidant who can't help but be truthful and have your best intentions in mind. The hardest thing for all of us to develop is that trust with ourselves, and we can strengthen it by practicing being *kind* to ourselves.

Choose a mantra. It can be anything from "I am beautiful" to "I radiate confidence and happiness because I choose to be confident, happy, and content with every aspect of myself" or anything in between. The only requirement is that the mantra must be kind and gentle, and it must hold enough truth that you don't have to call your own BS every time you say it.

My mantra of choice is "Today I am perfect." I like to include the immediacy of today because so often we get caught up worrying about the future or rehashing the past. We forget to live in the moment. It's easy to say we're going to enjoy the beauty of each day, but how often do we really stop to notice the splendor in the little things? The *natural* things. When we're at peace with ourselves, and when we befriend ourselves, we can begin to live in the now.

I chose the word *perfect* not because of the stigma of perfection in itself, but because to me the word embodies complete and utter contentedness. Things are never downright perfect, but shrugging off the imperfections and accepting them as part of the package allows us to focus only on the good. Whatever "perfection" means in my life changes every day, and waking up each morning and believing in my own true perfection is a breath of fresh air.

Choose a mantra that feels right (it could be anything!) and repeat it to yourself at a time of day that makes the most sense for you. I like to do it in the mornings when I'm getting ready because I'm already in front of the mirror and can really look into my eyes and hold myself accountable. Some people might prefer to recite their mantra during their morning commute or incorporate it into a bedtime ritual. Find what works for you and run with it.

The second trust-strengthening exercise is to practice *forgiveness* with yourself as much as possible. Say you lose your shit sitting in traffic or you spend an entire day completely obsessing over something that hasn't even happened yet. You are not a failure for doing either of those things. You are human! You are allowed to make mistakes. In fact, at the risk of sounding like a Hallmark card, the mistakes you make will actually strengthen your character as a whole and remind you why you make the choices you do.

So be your own best friend. Trust that chick or that dude you see in the mirror. Love that person. She/he rocks. A LOT. Believe it. Repeat that mantra until you are blue in the face if you need to, and forgive, forgive, forgive. And then start all over again because every friendship has its ups and downs, and the beauty of compassion and understanding is the foundation of any lasting relationship. Forgive yourself and befriend that awesome son of a gun.

BE KIND TO YOUR BODY BECAUSE YOU LOVE IT, NOT BECAUSE YOU HATE IT

Uh-oh, I said it. You were hoping I wasn't going to, but I totally just went there. "But Jordan, I don't love my body. That's why I'm reading this book . . . because I want to find balance and fall in love with myself!" Trust me, I get it. We have all been in a place where we feel completely unsatisfied with the way we look and feel, and we just want someone to point us in the right direction so we can change everything about ourselves from the ground up.

But believe me when I say that having that discontented mindset is our first mistake. We are setting ourselves up for failure before we've even made an inkling of a change. I'm not telling you that you have to go gaga for your love handles, your stretch marks, your cellulite, or your thigh chub in a way that means it's going to be there forever if you don't want it to, even though it's part of you and it *is* beautiful for that reason. I'm telling you that you have to love the body you reside in as a whole so you can make good choices for it when given the opportunity (which, um, inevitably will be every minute of every day).

Our bodies are our HOMES. Most of us are lucky enough to be able to bend, jump, leap, sweat, stretch, and run. Our bodies take us from A to B, they put up with all our nonsense, and they ward off sickness and disease on a daily basis. They are fine-tuned machines worthy of way more credit than they are usually given.

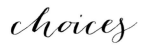

choices

"I'M TELLING YOU THAT YOU HAVE TO LOVE THE BODY YOU RESIDE IN AS A WHOLE SO YOU CAN MAKE GOOD CHOICES FOR IT WHEN GIVEN THE OPPORTUNITY (WHICH, UM, INEVITABLY WILL BE EVERY MINUTE OF EVERY DAY)."

If we make the choice to go for a two-mile (3.2 km) jog every day because we want to lose five pounds (2.3 kg), we're setting ourselves up for dissatisfaction. The first few days might feel like a breeze because the beginning of any new set of goals is accompanied by a jolt of adrenaline and determination. But when that first weigh-in comes around and we haven't lost as much as we'd wanted to, or we reach for a doughnut because we freaking feel like it, I am willing to bet we're going to get discouraged.

But if we make the choice to go for a two-mile (3.2 km) jog every day because we're appreciative of our body and everything it does for us, and because we want to get our hearts pumping so we can stay healthy and feel awesome, we're setting ourselves up for success. So what if you skip a day because you were tired or because you didn't want to miss a kickass birthday party? You can be grateful you ran the day before and you can trust yourself (see how that comes in? Tricky, TBB!) to run again when you can.

Positive goals lead to consistency. Consistency leads to trust. Trust leads to happiness, health and . . . you guessed it . . . balance!

EMBRACE YOUR DIFFERENCES INSTEAD OF COMPARING YOURSELF TO OTHERS

We've all done it. We've all seen that girl on the treadmill or that guy at the office who just seems to completely have their shit together. Their bod rocks, they ooze confidence, and their smile is so goddamn effortless we imagine their lives must be perfect. Actually, we take it a step further and daydream about this person's entire past, present, and future. They are probably madly in love with an equally hot spouse, have adorable kids, a successful job, a yacht in the South of France—the works.

There's nothing wrong with ogling someone who seems super cool and confident, as long as we keep a couple of things in mind. One, inevitably this person has their own insecurities and their own crap to deal with. It rocks that they have a smile on their face and a spring in their step because that's what we're all going for here anyway, right? Second, just because they have qualities we admire and perhaps desire does not mean that we don't have or can't work toward those qualities ourselves.

Instead of striving to be more like the people we admire, our time is better spent focusing on our strengths as individuals and working toward our own goals. For instance, I know I will never have long, lean Victoria's Secret model legs. I was born with short, athletic legs and strong, solid calves. I will never have a thigh gap, and short shorts will probably never be my best look.

So rather than lusting after Candice Swanepoel's runway gams, I focus on maintaining my muscle definition and working, stretching, and running my legs because it *feels* good and I enjoy doing it. There is no end goal other than health because I love my legs. They are my legs, and it is quite probable I will never have another pair! Similarly, I will never have the flat chest I dreamed about as an eighteen-year-old, and washboard abs are probably not going to pop out of my tummy in this lifetime.

Before I found my balance and fell in love with my body for the beauty of its abilities, I spent a lot of time comparing and contrasting my various parts to others I saw and thought looked good. I was never satisfied with my own results even though I was in great shape, and other than my stomach problems, I felt pretty great and healthy most of the time. All I have to say about that is I wasted a whole lot of time setting expectations for myself that actually had nothing to do with me as a person. If I achieved the legs or abs I thought I desired, I would only set a new goal and wouldn't even enjoy reaching the previous one. (I know this because I've reached my "goal weight" before and then some. The only thing that happened was that I created a new goal weight, one that was nearly impossible to attain.)

balance

"BEFORE I FOUND MY BALANCE AND FELL IN LOVE WITH MY BODY FOR THE BEAUTY OF ITS ABILITIES, I SPENT A LOT OF TIME COMPARING AND CONTRASTING MY VARIOUS PARTS TO OTHERS I SAW AND THOUGHT LOOKED GOOD."

In short, we do ourselves a major disservice by constantly comparing our bodies and lives to those people around us. I think it's okay and even healthy to set fitness and professional goals and draw inspiration from fit and successful people we admire. But when we lose sight of who we are and what we really want for ourselves, then we lose all ability to find balance.

Go back to your chosen mantra and remember to be kind to your body because you love it, not because you want it to look like someone else's. Remember that people out there are comparing themselves to YOU (seriously!) and wishing they could have what you have. Focus on the good and set goals you can work toward in a healthy and exciting way.

CONNECT WITH A HIGHER VERSION OF YOURSELF

I don't consider myself a religious person, but I do consider myself a spiritual person. My years of yoga and exploring the practices of karma and ahimsa (nonviolence) have brought me far closer to my spiritual self than my years in the temple studying for my Bat Mitzvah. I will always feel a connection to my Jewish heritage for communal and ancestral purposes, but as far as feeling the power of something beyond myself, I turn to yoga and meditation.

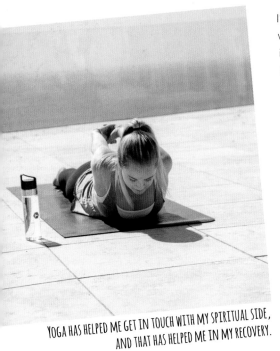

I'm willing to bet it has something to do with my extreme personality and my innate desire to practice rigorous exercise (type O blood, baby) and exert enough energy to exhaust myself before I can rest, but I feel closest to my spiritual self after working my body to the extreme in a hot yoga class or high intensity interval training (HIIT) session. After I channel my energy into movement, I can sit still, breathe, and turn inward.

It took me a long time to realize that the end of a yoga class served as a meditation practice for me. I knew that by the end of a class, I had usually worked myself up to a state of raw emotion and a feeling of blissful

YOGA HAS HELPED ME GET IN TOUCH WITH MY SPIRITUAL SIDE, AND THAT HAS HELPED ME IN MY RECOVERY.

peace with the universe, but I thought it was just the endorphins and the sweat talking. Being on the yoga mat helps me get out of my head for an hour and fifteen minutes, and that is a beautiful thing for an emotional loony tune like me. Once we can get out of our heads, we can lock into our minds without the noise of our everyday life. We can ponder the deeper meaning of things that plague us, and usually the answers we're seeking so desperately will start to come to us with ease.

Yoga and meditation don't work for everyone, but I am sharing my journey with them here because I do believe they work well for people with a tendency toward extremes. A simple bubble bath or back massage (although those are heavenly too!) isn't always going to cut it for us. A deep, inviting, spiritual practice with the vastly important quality of unhinging our minds from the everyday craziness can work wonders on the soul.

A truly balanced individual can channel an energy that is outside of his or her own body to deal with times of stress and even extreme happiness. It doesn't have to be as hippie-dippie as the meditation you might be imagining. You can even listen to a meditation podcast if that sounds like it would be up your alley. Plus, if you do, I'm willing to bet you'll sleep better too!

Find your yoga, whatever that may be. And for reference, yoga isn't just that bendy practice that requires major upper-body strength and an abundance of Lululemon clothing. *This* is what yoga is:

> "Yoga is the restraint of the modifications of the mind stuff."
> —YS 1.2 from Patanjali's *Yoga Sutras*

Try that one out on yourself next time you feel overwhelmed. Let me know how it goes.

spirituality

"A DEEP, INVITING, SPIRITUAL PRACTICE WITH THE VASTLY IMPORTANT QUALITY OF UNHINGING OUR MINDS FROM THE EVERYDAY CRAZINESS CAN WORK WONDERS ON THE SOUL."

CHALLENGE YOURSELF & TRY NEW THINGS

Balance, like knowledge, is an ever-evolving process. What balance meant to you last year isn't what it's going to mean to you today or even tomorrow. Allow yourself to advance and develop in new ways. We extreme-minded peeps are very susceptible to latching on to one routine or one label for all of time.

My veganism is a great example of something that once provided me wellness and balance and eventually stopped serving me in that way, but another, smaller-scale example is what I eat for breakfast. My breakfast balance has evolved over and over again and will continue to evolve for the rest of time. Sometimes a green smoothie is just what I need to fuel me through my morning and make me feel awesome, and sometimes the thought of drinking a tall glass of liquid in the a.m. sounds downright repulsive. Sometimes a smoothie *sounds* good, but I know I need something heavier to balance out a lighter dinner I may have had the night before. There was a period of time where gluten sent my stomach into gastrointestinal overdrive, but once in a while I can enjoy a slice of sourdough wheat walnut toast with almond butter and honey and feel fantastic. Sometimes eggs make me feel great, and sometimes they don't digest well at all.

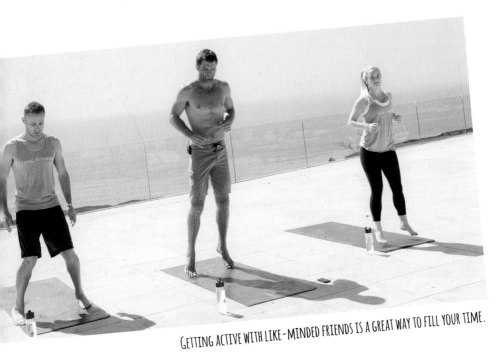

GETTING ACTIVE WITH LIKE-MINDED FRIENDS IS A GREAT WAY TO FILL YOUR TIME.

It's all about finding that balance and learning to listen to our bodies in order to fuel them in the best way. Beyond food, trying out new sports, hobbies, and even new poses in the yoga studio or exercises at the gym will open our eyes and might even capture our hearts as a new passion or favorite thing. Something I try to do on a weekly basis is hang out or at least connect with a new person who isn't in my close circle because *people* and their interactions with us have so much to teach us. There is a world of meaning behind a single conversation or even a single smile at a stranger (especially if it makes you uncomfortable to do it), and that meaning is what enhances our minds, bodies, and souls at the end of the day.

Write a list of challenges you want to accomplish within the next year. Don't be too overambitious, but it's not a bad idea to add a thing or two that terrifies the living daylights out of you. Trying new things can be awesome and exciting, and it can also be horrifying and uncomfortable. A good balance of both should ensure that your list is on the right track.

Depending on how goal-oriented you are, you can even set dates for accomplishing each goal. I am not a date-rigid person, which is why I gravitate toward the creative and relatively time-constraint-free blogging industry, but even setting a month or a season that you envision yourself finishing a goal is helpful in making sure you accomplish it.

Part of instilling and strengthening that trust in yourself means accomplishing the goals you set, so don't shrug your goals off for good just because you feel happy with your balance in the present moment. Allow yourself to evolve! Everything in the lifestyle is interconnected.

MAKE YOUR EVERYDAY LIFE FUN

I don't know if you're the type of person who finds grocery shopping boring or if you happen to find it insanely enjoyable like I do, but if it's a chore you dread, find ways to make it fun so you can incorporate it into your weekly or biweekly routine. That way, you will eat out less, dedicate yourself to making recipes that you enjoy and that also make you feel good, and you will spend more time enjoying yourself and less time doing things you feel like you're just "checking off the list."

Checking things off the list is what I call Robot Syndrome. Don't fall into it. If you're in it, pull yourself out of it. If you simply hate certain rituals like grocery shopping, dish washing, laundry folding, teeth brushing, and so on, find a way to make them more enjoyable. Do I sound like a total freak telling you to enjoy brushing your teeth if you've spent the last 893,439 hours of your life despising it?

Good. I am a freak. And I am here to make you a little more freaky and a little less robotic so you can get out of your head and leap into your balanced state of mind.

I, for one, detest taking showers. It's not that I am an unhygienic person. I actually shower just as much as everyone else I know, if not more often, because my hair looks totally dirty if I don't wash it every day. But I dread taking a shower each and every evening because that's twenty-ish minutes of time spent away from doing things I love like talking to people, working on the bloggy, writing, exercising, cooking, reading, and so on. And don't even get me started on the whole hair brushing and drying escapades and the occasional makeup application—such a dreadful routine!

But instead of viewing it that way (even though I obviously still have quite a ways to go to achieve complete balance here), I try to make my showering and getting ready routine more fun. I listen to music, I brainstorm blog post ideas, I massage my scalp while I wash and condition my hair (don't laugh at me; it feels good!), and I check in with myself about what else I need to do throughout the day and the week. And, if I remember, I practice my mantra.

The more we can make the little things fun, the less time we spend fretting and exuding unnecessary stress. Make a vow to have fun with yourself and change up your routine enough to enjoy the heck out of it!

freaky

"GOOD. I AM A FREAK. AND I AM HERE TO MAKE YOU A LITTLE MORE FREAKY AND A LITTLE LESS ROBOTIC SO YOU CAN GET OUT OF YOUR HEAD AND LEAP INTO YOUR BALANCED STATE OF MIND."

UNDERSTAND THE HEALTH BENEFITS OF FOODS YOU ENJOY

Knowledge is power. Research, learn, and understand the health benefits of fruits, veggies, and nutrient-dense foods. If you're eating food because it is nutrient-dense and because it will fuel you through your day and your workouts, you are much more likely to stay on track than if you're eating it to become a size 0. Similarly, eating to fuel your body versus eating to just "make the hunger go away" will strengthen your mind-body awareness and help hold you accountable for getting not only enough nutrients, but the right nutrients.

Similarly, research blood sugar and what you need to do to stabilize it and keep your cravings at bay. When we're in control of our bodies because we *understand* them, it feels amazingly powerful and has no correlation to restriction and unhealthy reasoning. Understand what your body needs so you can give yourself the gift of feeling amazing.

And if you really feel like you need an extra oomph to get going with your healthy lifestyle, you always have the option of seeing a nutritionist or health coach who can help you develop a tailored plan to meet your goals. (Cough, cough, you're looking at a health coach right here!)

GET YOUR FRIENDS INVOLVED

I do want you to be your own best friend, but I certainly don't want you to feel isolated or lonely. Surrounding yourself with awesome people is the cornerstone of all happiness and health. I realized not so long ago that the people in my life I feel closest to are kind of like extensions of myself. My family, my closest friends, and a few other kindred spirits fall into that category, and I am so unbelievably grateful for them. When I'm alone, I'm not fully alone. I have them, I can feel their energy, and it soothes me and makes me feel content no matter what is going on.

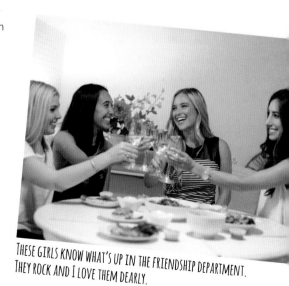

THESE GIRLS KNOW WHAT'S UP IN THE FRIENDSHIP DEPARTMENT. THEY ROCK AND I LOVE THEM DEARLY.

I know that my unusually strong attachment to the people I'm close to isn't something that everyone takes comfort in, but I am confident that surrounding ourselves with people we trust and admire is something we can all benefit from. And don't fret if you don't feel like you have a whole lot of people in your life who truly lift you up. Sometimes changing and evolving means outgrowing people we once got along great with and no longer do. It's never too late to find people to connect with, and there are so many amazing places to find them.

When you're in touch with your true and authentic self, you attract like-minded people. Once you get to that place, it will only be a matter of time before you start connecting with other people you get along with. Maybe you have similar interests, and maybe you couldn't be more different. Maybe there's a whole crew of eccentric personalities you rely on, or maybe there are a select few. If they make you feel good and bring positivity, then, they are keepers.

PAMPER YOURSELF

People make fun of me for taking extremely long bubble baths, but that's because being in the bathtub, surrounded by good-smelling candles and with a good book in hand, is one of my happiest happy places. I'm not going to deprive myself of the relaxation it gives me. When I have the time to take a bath and really enjoy it, I go all out. I stay in for hours, read, blast music, and soak and soak and soak.

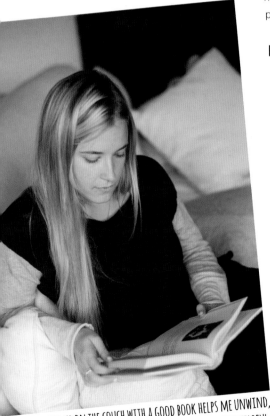

COZYING UP ON THE COUCH WITH A GOOD BOOK HELPS ME UNWIND, AND FINDING THAT STATE OF RELAXATION IS SO HELPFUL.

If you are the type of person to treat yourself with a cupcake or a beer at the end of a long workday, consider trying to treat yourself in ways that have nothing to do with food or alcohol. A stressful day can't be remedied by something outside of ourselves. In fact, believing it can is simply using food as a crutch to deal with something much larger. Relaxation techniques that come from within do us a whole lot more good than anything from the outside.

A monthly massage, weekly bubble bath, nightly walk, or even five minutes of reading before bed might be exactly what you need to address your nerves and unwind. If you still want a piece of chocolate or a glass of wine . . . go for it. Denying your cravings is never fun, and it usually leads to even more intensified cravings along with feelings of deprivation. But if you're going to feed your cravings, make sure to do it in a mindful way so you can enjoy the food or drink and let it satisfy you.

For many years, I satisfied my cravings because I knew it was "good" for me to do so, but that didn't help me from feeling guilty every time I ate a sugary treat or stayed out late drinking alcohol with friends. Now I do and eat whatever I please whenever it calls to me, and I do it because I *want* to and not because I feel like I should or because I'm using it to remedy a difficult day. It took me a *long* time to get there, and a lot of trial and error, but the important thing is that I got here.

Find what works for you and pamper yourself every single day like you would pamper a loved one on a special occasion. You deserve it! Balanced people don't apologize for squeezing the enjoyment out of every ounce of their lives.

INDULGE

As I mentioned above, indulge whenever you please. If you crave a brownie, ask yourself where the craving is coming from. Are you craving it because you've been stuck in traffic all afternoon and you're bored to tears, so eating chocolate sounds like way more fun than your current situation? Might you be craving it because your friend is stressing you out and you need to turn to something that feels comforting?

If the answer to that question leads you to something negative, you might want to continue exploring within before deciding what you really need. In my experience, cravings tend to crop up when my stomach is already upset about something else I've eaten. I feel like I might as well eat whatever sounds indulgent and delicious if my stomach is already full of acid and feeling yucky. That's never a good reason to indulge because I almost (okay, more than almost) always feel even worse after I do, since I'm not doing it for the right reasons.

Another way to prevent indulging at the wrong times is by asking yourself how you'll feel after you eat what you're craving. Will you feel satisfied and happy, or will you feel bloated and uncomfortable? Or maybe you'll feel a little overly full, but you're cool with that because it's a special occasion and you want the damn brownie. That's beyond fine too.

I spent way too long denying my every craving because no variation was allowed. My view was, "I didn't have a brownie yesterday, so I can't have one today. I don't eat refined sugar because it's bad for me, so obviously that means I will never, ever have it again even if I am starving and a sugary brownie is the last morsel on planet earth."

It was a pretty miserable way to live, and I don't miss anything about it. Now I take bites of anything that sounds good, and I don't feel obligated to eat the whole thing out of fear that it might be the very final time in my life I will allow myself to eat it.

Before you indulge, check in with yourself. Listen to your body. It knows the way, and you can be trusted to treat yourself without going overboard. I promise! If I can, you can.

allow

"NOW I TAKE BITES OF ANYTHING THAT SOUNDS GOOD, AND I DON'T FEEL OBLIGATED TO EAT THE WHOLE THING OUT OF FEAR THAT IT MIGHT BE THE VERY FINAL TIME IN MY LIFE I WILL ALLOW MYSELF TO EAT IT."

FIND THE BALANCE BETWEEN HEALTH AND RESTRICTION

Okay, this one is majorly important to me because I very much fell prey to it in the beginning of my eating disorder recovery. After living a super-strict plant-based vegan lifestyle for two years and restricting in various other ways before that, I felt like making healthy choices was a sin and emphasizing my health in any way would prevent me from recovering.

In actuality, that mentality was a reverse-eating-disorder voice in my mind that totally tripped me up in all the wrong ways. It's okay to be healthy. In fact, it's absolutely wonderful to be healthy. Focusing on nourishing our bodies with fresh, whole, organic foods from the earth is one way to rediscover a passion for feeling good and being kind to ourselves. Obsessing over healthy food like it's the only thing on this earth that has ever mattered, however, is not.

It can be very tough for us extreme beings to find a middle ground, especially if we've suffered from orthorexia or something similar. Recovering from orthorexia and maintaining my passion for health presented so, so many problems for me because often they stand in complete opposition to one another. My recovery voice told me to go for the burger instead of the kale salad, but my healthy voice reminded me that nothing is wrong with the kale salad and that I actually happen to love kale salads a lot of the time.

The difference is that finally, for once, I was not bound in chains to the kale salad. I could eat it because I wanted to eat it, which goes back to being in control of my own life and my decisions. It goes back to trusting myself. Similarly, I could totally eat the burger if I wanted to eat the burger. The extreme vacillation between the two and the panic and the obsession over making the choice are all the eating disorder. The eating and the decision making itself are the parts that should be enjoyable!

There is certainly a delicate balance between health and restriction, and we are more than allowed to be interested in health and make healthy choices because we enjoy them. That is not an eating disorder, it's a personal preference. And a healthy one at that!

KEEP A JOURNAL/FOOD JOURNAL

There have been times in my life when my journal is totally about the relationships with people in my life and other times when it is fully geared toward my relationship with food. I used to believe that a food journal and a personal, "stream of consciousness" journal had to be two completely separate things. Now I realize that to find my greatest level of balance, my regular journal and my food journal kind of blend into one, just like my regular thoughts and my food thoughts all blend into one. One is not more important or less important than the other. They simply are what they are.

A journal is a beautiful place to practice your mantra, to reflect on your meditation practice, and to set new goals. It is a safe, wonderful little object that can take on whatever role you'd like it to. It can be your BFF and confidant, or it can simply be a lettered list of awesome things that happened to you in a day or things you want to work on.

You can write in your journal as often or as little as you'd like, but I recommend keeping it consistent no matter how often you choose to update it. If you write in it every night, try to keep up that routine. If it's more of a Sunday night thing for you, then try to get to it every Sunday if you can. That way you can hold yourself accountable and check in with yourself on that deeper level that's harder to find when you're in the middle of your daily life.

ELIMINATE FOODS THAT MAKE YOU FEEL LIKE CRAP

Is this a scary one or what?! We see the word *eliminate* and we freak the heck out. Or if you're extreme and competitive like me, we see it and we get immediately intrigued. What can I eliminate that will make my life awesome and balanced and perfect and untainted forevermore?!

Umm, nothing. Sorry!

When I speak of elimination, I mean it in the broadest sense possible. Eliminate something for a constrained period of time and then reintroduce it if you so desire or continue to avoid it if it feels best in your body without it. If I hadn't cut out all different sorts of food groups in my plant-based days, I would never have known that now sometimes eggs make me feel a little funny and that I have to keep my dairy consumption to a minimum in order to feel my best.

I have also noticed after playing around with my diet that my body reacts differently to certain foods than it used to. I am now less sensitive to caffeine and gluten than I was before I avoided them completely for a few years, and I'm also a lot more sensitive to sugar than I used to be. Now it makes me hyper and jittery, whereas when I ate it on a very regular basis while growing up, I didn't even notice the effects it had on my mood, personality, or energy levels.

Playing with your diet in a healthy and nonjudgmental way is one great way to get to know your body from the inside out. I used to love juice cleanses for this reason, but now I believe in the power of solid-food "cleanses" that I prefer to call a reboot rather than a cleanse. I like to "reboot" by eating all fresh, plant-based food for a few days or even a half day at a time when I'm feeling bogged down and like I need to connect to a healthier way of life.

I don't get crazy about it like I once did. I add in some fish if I feel like it, and I have a few bites of chocolate if it's calling my name. I spent two years avoiding anything that wasn't part of the "plan," otherwise known as the vegan label, like the absolute plague. It was not healthy because I was doing it for all the wrong reasons. Now when I choose to pay attention to the foods I'm putting into my body, I do it in a mindful way and because I love my body, not because I hate it or because I'm mad at it for having digestion problems or for any other silly, illegitimate reason.

elimination

"WHEN I SPEAK OF ELIMINATION, I MEAN IT IN THE BROADEST SENSE POSSIBLE. ELIMINATE SOMETHING FOR A CONSTRAINED PERIOD OF TIME AND THEN REINTRODUCE IT IF YOU SO DESIRE OR CONTINUE TO AVOID IT IF IT FEELS BEST IN YOUR BODY TO DO THAT."

Foods I've found beneficial to eliminate for days or weeks at a time are dairy, wheat, red meat, refined sugar, and processed food. Depending on your level of health and your experience with cutting foods out of your diet, you can try eliminating foods you think might trigger not feeling well. You can do it all at once, if you're seasoned with this sort of thing, or you can do them one at a time. If a serious elimination diet interests you, I suggest finding a health coach or nutritionist to work with to help you tailor the plan to fit your needs and goals. We are all so very different, remember that!

SEE YOURSELF THROUGH A STRANGER'S EYES

One of the saddest things about living in this image-driven world of ours is that we can be entirely perfect and beautiful in a stranger's eyes, but in our own eyes we pick ourselves apart. No matter how healthy and fit we may be, we are always going to pick out the one thing about ourselves that we don't like. And if we fix that, we will be on to the next issue.

We should all challenge ourselves to let those self-judgments go. I pose this test to you: View yourself through *someone else's eyes*. Look at yourself as the stranger in the yoga room sees you, or the girl on the sidewalk, or the new coworker you haven't gotten the chance to know yet. See yourself from the eyes of a stranger, a loved one, or an old friend. See it all. Tell yourself you can be the person someone else sees you to be, because you're *happy*, healthy, friendly, and confident—not because you have a perfect body or eat a perfect diet.

Next time you look in the mirror, I challenge you to pretend you're seeing yourself for the first time. Pretend you have one shot to make an impression on yourself. How would you carry yourself? What would you want to see?

happy

"TELL YOURSELF YOU CAN BE THE PERSON SOMEONE ELSE SEES YOU TO BE, BECAUSE YOU'RE *HAPPY*, HEALTHY, FRIENDLY, AND CONFIDENT—NOT BECAUSE YOU HAVE A PERFECT BODY OR EAT A PERFECT DIET."

DON'T TAKE YOURSELF TOO SERIOUSLY

Hands down the best cure for the soul and for the pain of imbalance is to allow yourself to be SILLY! Be a freak. Be a total, godforsaken, out of this world, lighthearted dork of all dorkiness. Speak your mind and say whatever the heck you feel like saying. Forget about the filter you've turned on to make yourself a socially acceptable being. Be you. Be cray-cray.

The people who know me best, and I mean know me *really* well, know I am a total oddball. There isn't a cool bone in my body, and I like it that way. There were a whole lot of years when I thought I was super cool because I felt I could "fit in" with just about any crowd, but at the end of the day that didn't really serve me. Instead it led to me doing things I didn't really care to do and to an eventual disconnection between my mind and my body and ultimately my spiritual self.

I surround myself with people who love me unconditionally, and I love them right back. I don't waste my time with people who I feel judged by or who I see judging others in a way I don't agree with. I give people second, third, and fourth chances because I very much believe most people have a unique and remarkable friendship to offer, but if I don't feel the connection, then I don't waste my time forcing it.

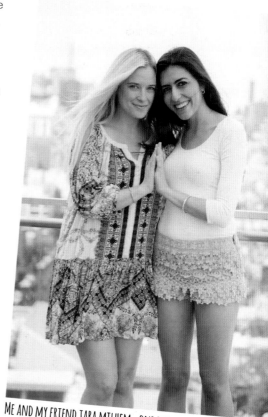

I don't take myself very seriously (at all), and I encourage others to do the same. Sometimes I get sleepy and hyper and hungry and tongue-tied all at the same time. And you know what? Some of my most enjoyable moments spawn out of those moods.

If there are people in your life who make you feel confined in a box that no longer serves you, it's okay to move away from them and eventually

ME AND MY FRIEND TARA MILHEM , ONE OF THOSE INCREDIBLE FRIENDS WHO MAKES LIFE SO MUCH MORE FUN.

cut ties if that's what your heart tells you to do. Surround yourself with people who support you and help you step into your light—people around whom you're comfortable being your truest, weirdest, and most real self.

DON'T TAKE THIS LIST TOO SERIOUSLY

At one point in my life, if someone was offering me a guide toward a balanced lifestyle, I would have etched the principles onto my arm in blood and abided by them as if they were the word of God. (Just kidding on the blood part . . . but only kinda.) Part of leading a balanced life means picking and choosing what works for you, what excites you, and what makes the most sense for you. If you're feeling totally lost, and a strong sense of direction is what you're looking for right now, then by all means follow this list down to a T. Inscribe it on your bedroom wall and check things off your goal list like there's no tomorrow! (This is probably what I would do if I were reading a list like this, by the way.)

But if you feel like you've already begun to develop a firm grasp on what balance means to you, then trust yourself to decide which principles you can draw inspiration from right now. They might be different from what you're looking for tomorrow, next week, or next year. Check in with yourself often to make sure you're propelling yourself forward and maintaining your version of balance.

You can do it. I have more faith in you than you can imagine.

Let's do this!

16

THE BALANCED RECIPE GUIDE

Welcome! These recipes are meant to guide you toward a happy, healthy, and delicious relationship with food centered on a diet full of fresh foods from the earth. Playing around with different types of vegetables, fruit, grains, fish, poultry, and legumes in the kitchen helped me fall in love with variety in my meals again. Learning to bring out their natural flavors with simple and whole ingredients reminded me that food is meant not only for fuel but also enjoyment. The act of preparing the food is just as important as the act of eating it.

It is a total myth that orthorexia and healthy food are one in the same. In fact, an important step in recovery from any eating disorder is realizing and embracing the beauty of food as medicine. When we fuel our bodies with food that nourishes our body, mind, and soul, we have no choice but to begin to develop a healthy, symbiotic relationship with what we put into our mouths. Cooking is such a healing and fun part of the process of finding what works for our bodies, and it is part of our personal journey to find what we like and what we don't like. Make it fun, and keep the pressure out of it!

These recipes are meant to be simple. Many of us live busy, active lives and don't have time to be full-time chefs. All of these recipes will take you less than an hour to prepare (most even much less than that) and can be adapted for a party of one or an entire group. I hope you enjoy playing around with them as much as I have, and don't forget: we all feel our best when we treat our bodies like they deserve to be treated. Have your kale, and have your (healthy, usually) dessert, too.

Chocolate & Greens
JAR OF YUMMINESS

Jars of Yumminess (aka JOY) are my go-to. Layered, colorful, nutrient-rich blended oats, they were one of the first recipes to appear on the blog. I still make JOY whenever I find the time, and the great thing about them is they're packed with about quadruple the amount of oatmeal I would normally eat for breakfast, so I get to enjoy them for a whole week straight when I do!

FOR THE OATS:
2 cups (160 g) dry oats,
   gluten-free, if necessary
2 cups (475 ml) almond milk
2 cups (475 ml) water

FOR THE GREEN PORTION:
1 teaspoon spirulina
1 handful of fresh spinach

FOR THE CHOCOLATE PORTION:
1 to 2 tablespoons (5 to 10 g)
   raw cacao powder
2 tablespoons (22 g) dairy-free
   chocolate chips or (16 g) raw
   cacao nibs

**FOR THE RAW CHOCOLATE SAUCE
(OPTIONAL):**
⅓ cup (75 g) coconut oil, melted
½ cup (40 g) raw cacao powder

FOR THE TOPPINGS:
½ of a ripe banana
1 tablespoon (11 g) dairy-free
   chocolate chips or (8 g) raw
   cacao nibs
¼ cup (28 g) slivered almonds

To make the oats: Boil the oats in the almond milk and water until the liquid is fully absorbed, about 15 to 20 minutes.

To make the green portion: Combine half of the cooked oats with the spirulina and spinach and blend in a blender or food processor until thoroughly combined. Layer ½ cup (115 g) at the bottom of a jar, glass, or bowl. Set the excess ½ cup (115 g) aside for now.

To make the chocolate portion: Combine the remaining cooked oats with the cacao powder and blend until thoroughly combined. If you want your chocolate oats to be thicker, use a spoon to mix them instead of a blender. Once blended, add the chocolate chips or cacao nibs and stir until thoroughly combined. Layer ½ cup (115 g) on top of the green portion.

Layer the second ½ cup (115 g) of the green portion on top of the chocolate oats. Then layer the second ½ cup (115 g) of the chocolate portion on top of the green oats.

Top with sliced banana, chocolate chips or cacao nibs and slivered almonds. Drizzle with optional raw chocolate sauce. Enjoy!

Yield: 4 servings

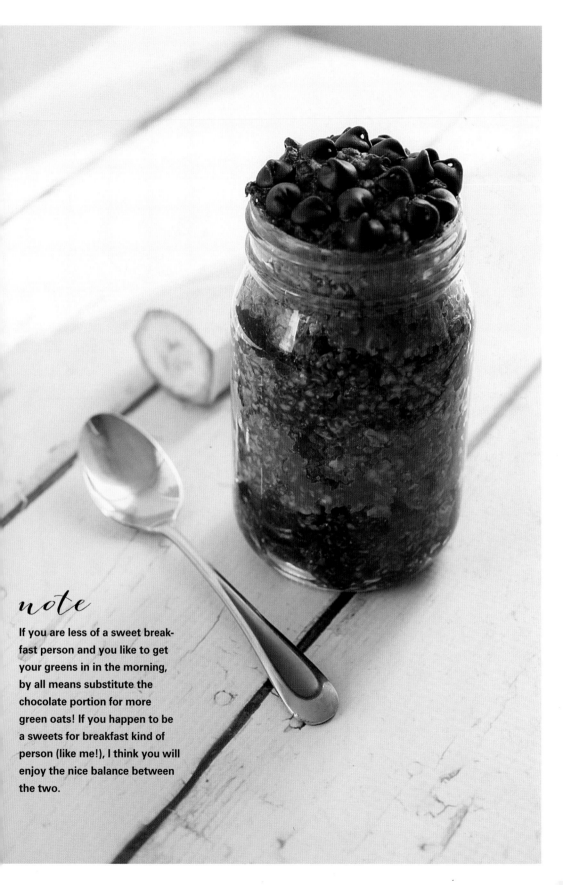

note

If you are less of a sweet breakfast person and you like to get
your greens in in the morning,
by all means substitute the
chocolate portion for more
green oats! If you happen to be
a sweets for breakfast kind of
person (like me!), I think you will
enjoy the nice balance between
the two.

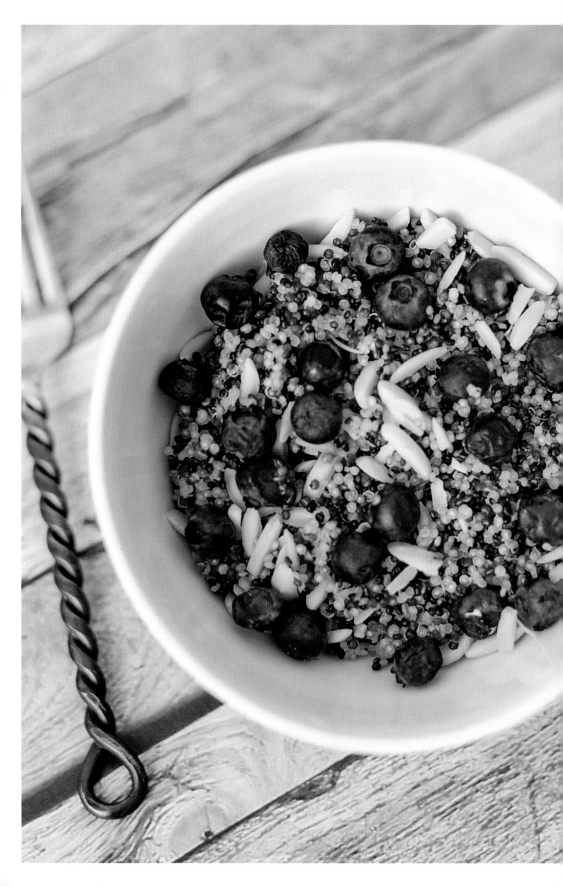

Warm Quinoa BREAKFAST CEREAL

Swapping your usual oatmeal or sugary cereal in the morning for a bowl of nutty quinoa can give you an extra boost of protein and fiber, and for us gluten-free folks, it can be a great warming breakfast that might otherwise seem hard to find sans gluten (e.g., oatmeal, toast, pancakes, french toast, you know the rest). I love adding a splash of almond milk into my quinoa to give it a real cereal vibe. Who doesn't remember those weekend mornings as a kid, sitting on the couch watching cartoons and digging into a bowl of cereal and milk?! The blueberries give it a sweet zing, while the cinnamon brings out the natural flavors and turns our typically savory quinoa dish into a sweet one. This might just become your new breakfast go-to.

½ cup (87 g) uncooked quinoa
1½ cups (355 ml) water
A few pinches of cinnamon
1 teaspoon honey, optional (You may substitute agave syrup, maple syrup, liquid stevia, or coconut sugar.)
½ cup (120 ml) almond milk
¼ cup (36 g) blueberries
¼ cup (28 g) slivered almonds

Cook the quinoa in the water over medium-high heat until the quinoa has absorbed the water, about 15 to 20 minutes. Fluff with a fork and pour into a bowl.

Stir in the cinnamon and the optional sweetener.

Pour in the almond milk and top with blueberries and slivered almonds.

Yield: 1 serving

note

I love adding a few drops of liquid stevia to this dish when I am trying to start my day with stabilized blood sugar levels. In the beginning of my recovery process, it was hard for me to keep my blood sugar levels in check, so swapping honey and agave syrup with liquid stevia helped me maintain my satiety longer and keep my sugar cravings at bay. It's all natural, and it's great stuff. I highly recommend looking into it!

CREAMY MACA *Buckwheat* PORRIDGE

One fabulous thing that my vegan days left me with is a love for soaked anything. I soak away, all the time, because it's so good for our digestion to soak certain ingredients in water and let their natural enzymes release. Soaking also makes proteins more readily available and eradicates toxins. I soak oats, nuts, seeds, and even buckwheat groats.

What are buckwheat groats, you ask? I asked the same thing when I came across a recipe for raw buckwheat porridge on a raw foods blog I followed back in the day. Buckwheat groats are the hulled seeds of the buckwheat plant, otherwise known as a mild-tasting, nutty, oat-like flavored grain. They are also nutritional powerhouses. You won't regret trying them!

½ cup (78 g) buckwheat groats, soaked overnight

1 very ripe banana

1 teaspoon tahini (You can also use a nut butter variation.)

2 teaspoons maca*

1 teaspoon raw cacao powder*

1 date, pitted

¼ cup (60 ml) almond milk (or any nut milk variation)

FOR THE TOPPINGS:
I used a handful of blueberries, coconut meat, and cacao nibs for topping, but anything will do!

Soak the buckwheat groats overnight in 1 to 2 cups of water.

Combine the soaked buckwheat, banana, tahini, maca, cacao, date, and nut milk into a blender or food processor and blend until smooth and creamy. Pour into a bowl, and top with your desired toppings. Enjoy.

Yield: 2 servings

note

If you don't have these fancy superfoods, you can do without them and just add more nut butter, nut milk, and some spices, such as cinnamon and/or nutmeg!

LOW-GLYCEMIC GREEN
Smoothie DELICIOUSNESS

I got into the whole low-glycemic smoothie thing once I realized that the less sugar I consumed in the morning via fruit in my smoothies, the more sugar I could eat later on in the form of a healthy dessert without feeling too over-sugared! It's all about balance, right? I also love the way it feels to pack my body with healthy, nutrient-dense fats in the morning and let that energy fuel me through until lunch. Plus, with the cacao powder and the mint leaves, this still tastes like a healthified version of a mint chip smoothie!

1 cup (30 g) spinach or (67 g) kale
¼ cup (36 g) blueberries
¼ avocado, pitted and peeled
1 tablespoon (10 g) chia seeds
1 tablespoon (5 g) cacao powder
1 handful fresh mint leaves
1 cup (235 ml) almond milk
½ cup ice

Place all ingredients into a high-speed blender, and blend until smooth.

Yield: 1 serving

SUGAR-FREE *Pumpkin* SPICE SMOOTHIE

This smoothie can be enjoyed as a dessert, a meal, or an afternoon snack—that's the beauty of being sugar-free and full of nutrients! Also, canned pumpkin puree is available year-round, so if you happen to be craving a Halloween-esque meal midsummer, you know I've got you covered. The cinnamon in this makes it an extra-tasty treat, and sometimes I even like to blend in a bit of vanilla bean!

½ cup (123 g) pumpkin puree
1 cup (30 g) fresh spinach or
   kale (67 g)
1 tablespoon (16 g) almond butter
1 cup (235 ml) almond milk
½ cup (109 g) ice
A few pinches of cinnamon
1 scoop of plant-based protein
   powder, optional (I like either
   chocolate or vanilla Vega One.)

Blend all the ingredients thoroughly and enjoy!

Yield: 1 serving

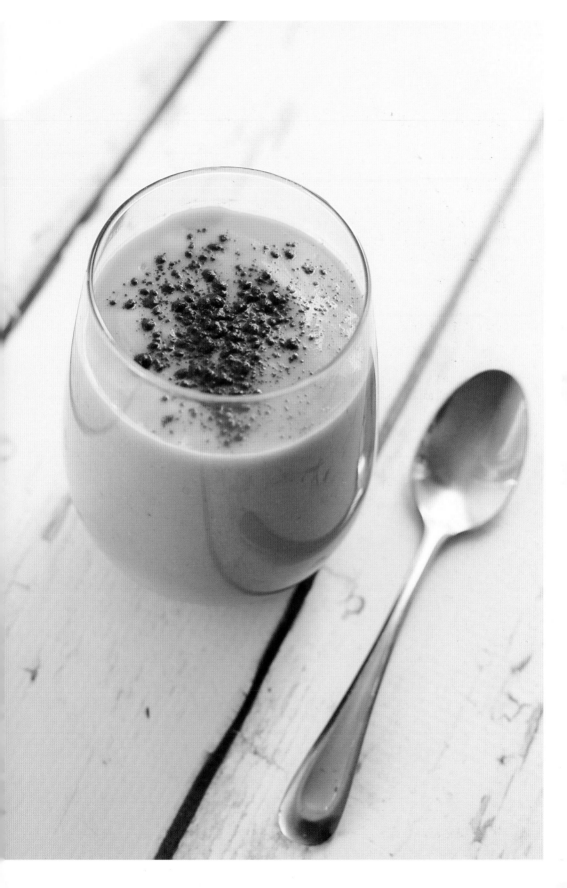

THE BALANCED SMOOTHIE

To combat the craziness (and stomachache) that sometimes comes from running wild with smoothie ingredients and combinations, I developed this simple green smoothie recipe. Even if I decide to switch it up, I use it as my base. And it has definitely won over my not-so-sure-about-this-smoothie-business friends and family! "Wait, will you make me that one smoothie again? You know, the one in the mason jar that you took a hundred photos of." It's music to my ears!

1 overripe banana
1 cup (30 g) fresh spinach or (67 g) kale
½ cup (75 g) blueberries
1 tablespoon (16 g) almond butter
½ cup (120 ml) almond milk
½ cup (120 ml) water
½ cup (109 g) ice
1 scoop of plant-based protein powder, optional

Blend all the ingredients thoroughly and enjoy!

Yield: 1 serving

TROPICAL SMOOTHIE

One rule: Kick back and pretend you are on a tropical vay-cay while drinking this one! And maybe put in a little toothpick umbrella if you have one. (Okay, that's two rules.)

1 cup (187 g) frozen diced mango
1 cup (30 g) fresh spinach
½ cup (48 g) fresh mint leaves
½ cup (120 ml) coconut water
½ cup (120 ml) water
½ cup (109 g) ice

Blend all the ingredients thoroughly and enjoy!

Yield: 1 serving

BAKED *Carrot Cake* OATMEAL

Baked oatmeal has got to be one of my favorite ways to enjoy breakfast. I love that this recipe incorporates veggies (carrots), protein (walnuts), and fiber (oats). I always try to make sure my meals are as balanced as possible, and that's easy to do with this one. I like to keep it tummy-friendly and gluten-free by using gluten-free oats, but if you prefer to use a different kind, then be my guest!

Coconut oil or butter

1 cup (80 g) rolled oats (gluten-free, if necessary)

1 teaspoon cinnamon

1 teaspoon baking powder

1 cup (110 g) shredded carrots

1 cup (235 ml) almond milk (or milk of choice)

1 teaspoon of freshly grated ginger

¼ cup (30 g) chopped walnuts

Preheat the oven to 375°F (190°C, gas mark 5) and lightly grease a small baking dish with coconut oil or butter.

In a large bowl, mix together the oats, cinnamon, and baking powder.

In a separate bowl, whisk together the carrots, almond milk, and ginger.

Pour the carrot, almond milk, and ginger mixture over the oat mixture and mix thoroughly. Transfer to the baking dish and smooth it out with a spoon. Sprinkle the walnuts on top and bake for 30 to 35 minutes or until lightly browned along the edges.

Let it cool and enjoy. It's also great for leftovers!

Yield: 1 to 2 servings

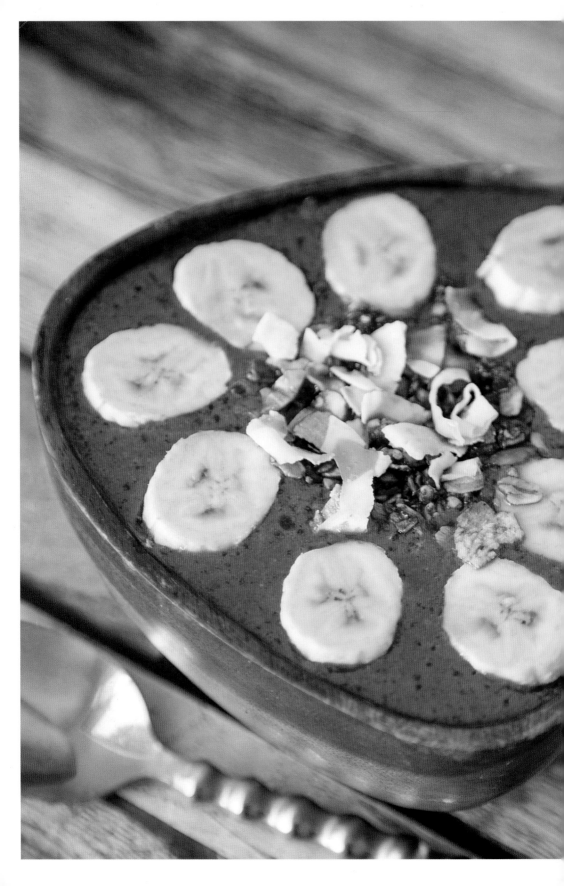

Simple Superfood ACAI BOWL

I am freakishly into acai bowls. And I know what you're thinking: The obsessive girl is freakishly into something—greaaattt. But not to worry! I didn't touch acai bowls with a ten-foot pole when I was suffering from orthorexia, I'm sad to say, because even though I warned others not to fear the sugar content in fruit, I totally fell prey to counting grams of sugar and getting compulsive. Now I enjoy acai bowls whenever I feel like having them and especially the healthiest variations that I make for myself. I'm sharing my super-healthy, simple, and delicious acai bowl recipe with *you* because it's packed full of superfoods, antioxidants, fiber, and deliciousness. I hope you love it as much as I do!

FOR THE ACAI BOWL:

1 overripe banana

2 tablespoons (9 g) acai powder
  or 1 packet (100 g, or 3.5 oz)
  frozen acai

1 tablespoon (5 g) cacao powder

1 tablespoon (15 g) maca powder

1 tablespoon (16 g) almond butter

A few pinches of cinnamon

FOR THE TOPPINGS:

½ cup (75 g) blueberries

½ of a banana, thinly sliced

¼ cup (31 g) granola (gluten-free,
  if neccessary)

1 tablespoon (4 g) coconut flakes

Blend all of the ingredients and pour into a bowl. Top with the toppings and enjoy! It's super simple.

Yield: 1 to 2 servings

note

I know this recipe has some funky superfoods in it (namely, cacao and maca powder), and if you don't have them on hand in your kitchen, don't be afraid! This bowl will still be delicious and packed full of nutrients without them. If you want to try them, they are available online and in many health food stores. Cacao is a great antioxidant for natural, sustained energy and destroying free radicals. Maca is rich in vitamins B, C, and E and also provides plenty of zinc, magnesium, iron, and amino acids. These babies are nutrient powerhouses!

GREEN MACHINE JUICE

In the past few years, juicing has morphed from a trend in the health food community into somewhat of a universal obsession—probably because juices are such an easy and delicious way to pack so many nutrients into your body. And as long as you don't take it overboard and start replacing your meals with juices, then juicing is a great choice to make in my book.

---

1 green apple, halved
2 stalks of celery
1 cucumber
5 kale leaves
½ of a lemon, peeled
1 inch (2.5 cm) piece of fresh ginger

Process the green apple, celery, cucumber, kale, lemon, and ginger through a juicer. If you don't have a juicer, you can use a blender, but you will want to add about ½ cup (120 ml) water and some ice.

Pour into a glass and enjoy.

Yield: 1 serving

LEMON-CAYENNE JUICE

You might find this recipe similar to the recipe for the original Master Cleanse drink—just be excited that you are not fasting on this and *only* this for days or weeks on end. The agave syrup and cayenne will give you an energy boost, while the lemon will soothe your digestive system and cleanse the colon. This juice doesn't have a lot of protein, carbohydrates, fats, or minerals (that's why the Master Cleanse is not sustainable for long periods of time), but it's the perfect supplement to the rest of the meals you will nourish yourself with today.

---

8 ounces (235 ml) water
Juice of ¼ of a lemon
Pinch of cayenne pepper
1 tablespoon (20 g) agave syrup

Blend the ingredients thoroughly and enjoy!

Yield: 1 serving

SOUTHWESTERN BAKED *Sweet Potato*

I can't seem to eat a baked potato without wanting to "load it up" with all the yummy fixings. I blame it on my childhood trips to Sun Valley, Idaho—the home of the original baked potato loaded with melty cheese, butter, sour cream, chives, and bacon bits. However delicious it was while I ate it, that stuffed potato always left my tummy reeling later on. Because I wasn't willing to give up my savory favorite, I decided I was going to make a healthy, nutrient-packed, and tummy-friendly version. Enter the Southwestern Baked Sweet Potato.

FOR THE POTATO:

1 large sweet potato

½ cup (83 g) cubed tempeh

1 teaspoon olive oil

2 tablespoons (14 g) ground cumin

¼ cup (60 g) canned black beans, drained

¼ cup (53 g) canned corn, drained

4 sliced cherry tomatoes

FOR THE AVOCADO-CILANTRO SAUCE:

1 ripe avocado

1 clove of garlic

½ cup (8 g) fresh cilantro

Juice of ½ of a lime

¼ cup (60 ml) water (Add more or less depending on the texture you're going for.)

2 tablespoons (14 g) ground cumin

Salt and pepper, to taste

Preheat the oven, to 350°F (180°C, gas mark 4).

Bake the sweet potato for about 45 minutes to an hour or until soft. You can test the softness by poking a fork through the top.

Slice the tempeh into cubes, lay them on a baking sheet, and pour the olive oil and cumin over them.

Bake the tempeh along with the sweet potato for about 20 minutes or until golden brown and crispy.

To make the avocado-cilantro sauce: Blend the avocado, garlic, cilantro, lime juice, water, and cumin. Taste and then add more water, salt, and pepper if necessary to reach your desired taste and consistency. You will have some left over!

Once the potato is fully baked, slice it down the middle and remove a large spoonful from the center. Add the desired amount of the avocado-cilantro sauce, black beans, corn, tomatoes, and tempeh.

Top with salt or extra cumin and lime juice to taste.

Yield: 1 to 2 servings

Macho Chicken CHOPPED SALAD

This salad is an adaptation from my favorite restaurant in the whole wide world called Bandera. It's in my hometown of Sacramento, but when I moved to Los Angeles, I learned that there are Banderas scattered around Southern California as well! For a couple of years, I couldn't order anything at Bandera except for the seasonal veggie plate with no oil and no Parmesan, but when I transitioned back into a balanced diet, I was finally able to order the Macho Salad again. The salad boasts the perfect combo of protein, veggies, crunch, and sweetness. It's only my favorite kind of meal. This is *The Balanced Blonde*'s twist on Bandera's original.

FOR THE SALAD:
1 cup (55 g) mixed salad greens
1 cup (30 g) fresh spinach
1 cup (238 g) shredded chicken
3 dates, pitted and chopped
½ cup (105 g) canned corn, drained
½ cup (75 g) chopped cherry tomatoes
¼ cup (25 g) halved walnuts
½ of an avocado
¼ cup (38 g) crumbled goat cheese

FOR THE LEMON VINAIGRETTE:
2 tablespoons (28 ml) extra virgin
  olive oil
4 tablespoons (60 ml) freshly
  squeezed lemon juice
1 tablespoon (10 g) crushed garlic
½ teaspoon Dijon mustard
Salt and pepper, to taste

To make the salad: Combine all of the salad ingredients in a bowl and mix well.

To make the lemon vinaigrette: Combine all of the ingredients in a small bowl and mix thoroughly. If you like your salad dressing thicker, add more mustard. If you prefer a lighter dressing, add more lemon juice.

Pour the dressing over the salad and toss until well combined. Enjoy!

Yield: 2 servings

note

If you are trying to limit your sugar intake for health reasons or preferences, substitute the dates with fresh blueberries or omit. If you want to make this dairy-free without losing the creamy texture of the cheese, add hummus or tahini.

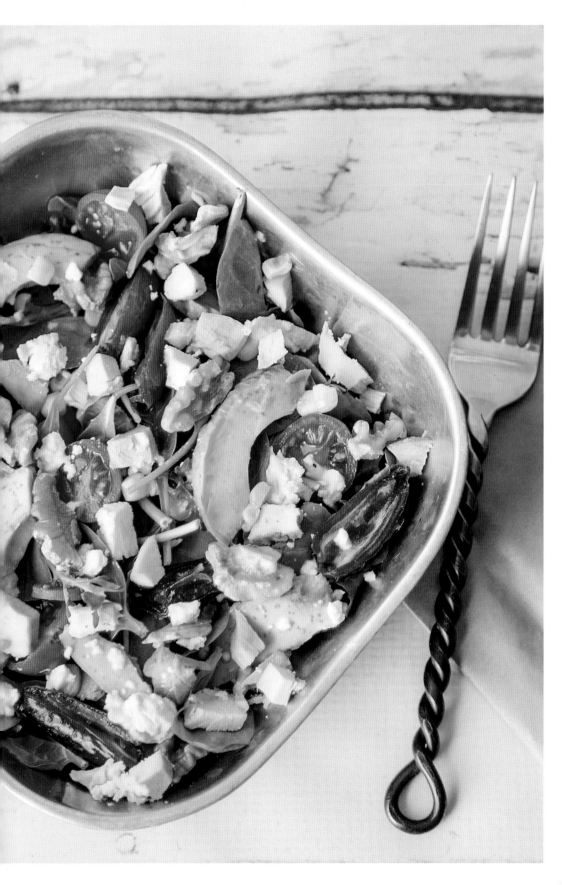

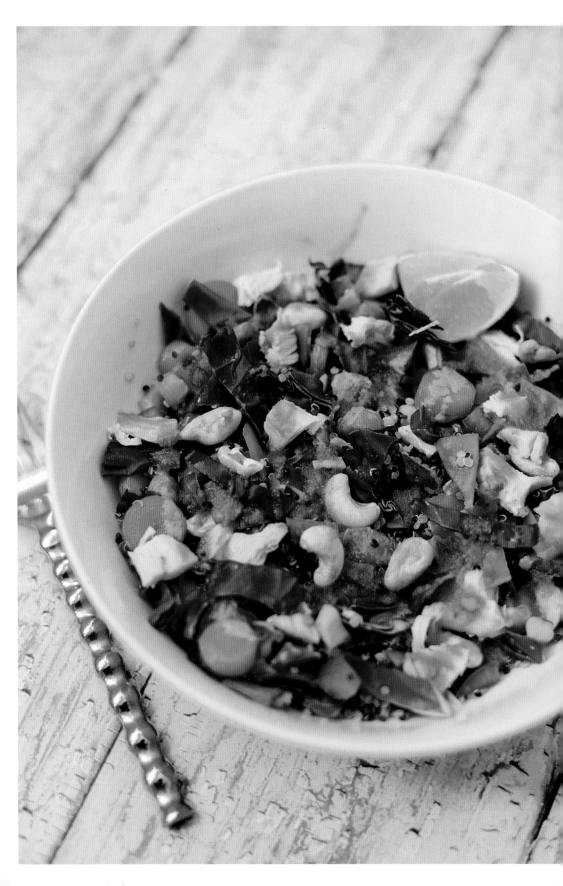

Cashew Crunch THAI QUINOA SALAD

Thai food has got to be my favorite cuisine in the universe, especially because the tangy and sweet combo in Thai dishes makes my taste buds do a little happy dance. The only problem with most food at Thai restaurants is the abundance of butter, sodium, and oil used. Homemade Thai is the way to go for a balanced diet and a happy tummy! (That's most of the time, of course.) Plus, the cashews in this salad make for a super-crunchy surprise in every bite.

FOR THE QUINOA SALAD:
1 cup (173 g) uncooked quinoa
3 cups (700 ml) water
1 cup (166 g) cubed chicken
1 to 2 tablespoons (15 to 28 ml) sesame oil
2 cups (140 g) shredded red cabbage
1 green bell pepper, diced
1 cup (110 g) shredded carrots
¼ cup (25 g) sliced scallions
½ cup (75 g) shelled edamame
½ cup (70 g) cashew halves
Fresh lime

FOR THE DRESSING:
¼ cup (60 g) all-natural tahini (ground sesame seeds)
¼ cup (65 g) peanut butter
2 tablespoons (28 ml) low-sodium soy sauce or liquid aminos
1 tablespoon (20 g) honey (You may substitute agave syrup or [9 g] coconut palm sugar.)
1 tablespoon (15 ml) rice vinegar
1 teaspoon coconut oil
2 tablespoons (28 ml) water
2 teaspoons freshly grated ginger, optional

To make the quinoa salad: Cook the quinoa in the water over medium-high heat until the quinoa has absorbed the water, about 15 to 20 minutes. Fluff with a fork and set aside.

Sauté the chicken in the sesame oil in a saucepan over medium-high heat until golden brown.

Chop and dice all the vegetables and nuts and fold into the quinoa. Add the chicken and stir until the mixture is well combined.

To make the dressing: Melt the tahini and peanut butter in a microwave-safe bowl or over medium-high heat on a stovetop, if necessary. Combine all the sauce ingredients in the bowl and stir until smooth.

Top the salad with the dressing and garnish with a lime to taste. (I love the tanginess.) Serve warm or chilled. (The flavors are even better the next day.)

Yield: 4 servings

note

If you are a cilantro person, cilantro and extra chopped cashews make a beautiful and delicious addition to this salad as well.

Chicken Teriyaki BOWL

I love eating my food in bowls. In fact, I love it so much, I often pour things into bowls that most people would eat on a plate or simply with their hands. My favorite thing to do is combine a medley of yummy, balanced flavors in a bowl and enjoy how the flavors complement each other. This tangy, zesty, and über-healthy Chicken Teriyaki Bowl does just that. It's the healthier version of your typical Chinese restaurant chicken teriyaki—and it's just as delicious, I promise. (What do you take me for?!)

FOR THE BOWL:
6 ounces (170 g) chicken breast
1 tablespoon (15 ml) light olive oil
  or (14 g) coconut oil, melted
½ cup (95 g) brown rice
1 cup (235 ml) water
¼ cup (25 g) diced scallions
1 cup (71 g) chopped broccoli florets

FOR THE TERIYAKI SAUCE:
½ cup (120 ml) organic soy sauce
1½ tablespoons (30 g) maple syrup
¼ teaspoon ginger
¼ teaspoon garlic
½ tablespoon arrowroot powder

Preheat the oven to 450°F (230°C, gas mark 8).

To make the bowl: Drizzle the chicken with the olive oil or coconut oil and bake in the oven for about 20 minutes or until cooked through but still juicy.

Boil the rice in the water over medium-high heat for about 30 minutes or until the water is fully absorbed, stirring occasionally. I like to add more water while it cooks to make it as fluffy as can be.

To make the teriyaki sauce: In a small saucepan, heat all the teriyaki ingredients on low for about 7 minutes or until the mixture starts to bubble. Transfer to a sealed container. I use a mason jar.

Throw the scallions and spinach into a small saucepan with a dash of coconut oil or olive oil. Sauté for 3 to 5 minutes or until golden brown.

Place the rice, greens, and chicken into a bowl and spoon the teriyaki sauce over it. Enjoy!

Yield: 1 to 2 servings

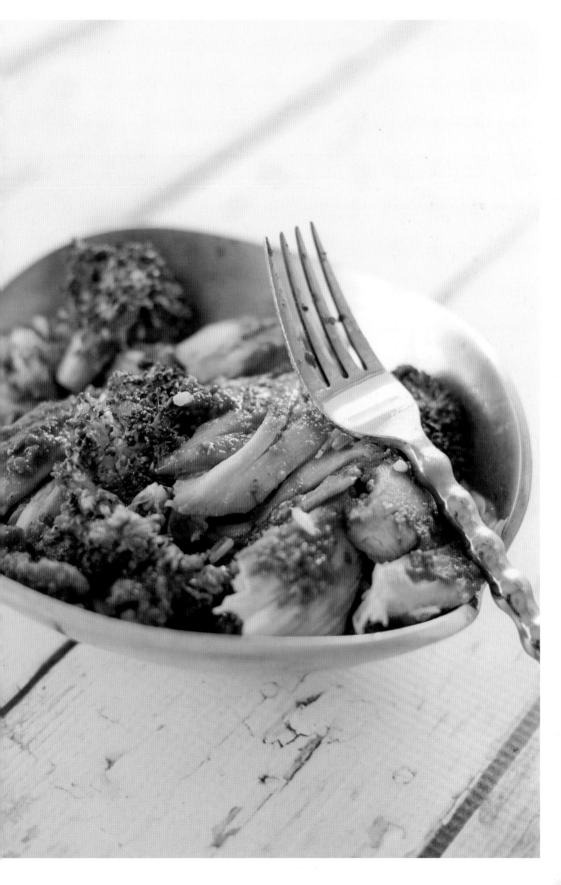

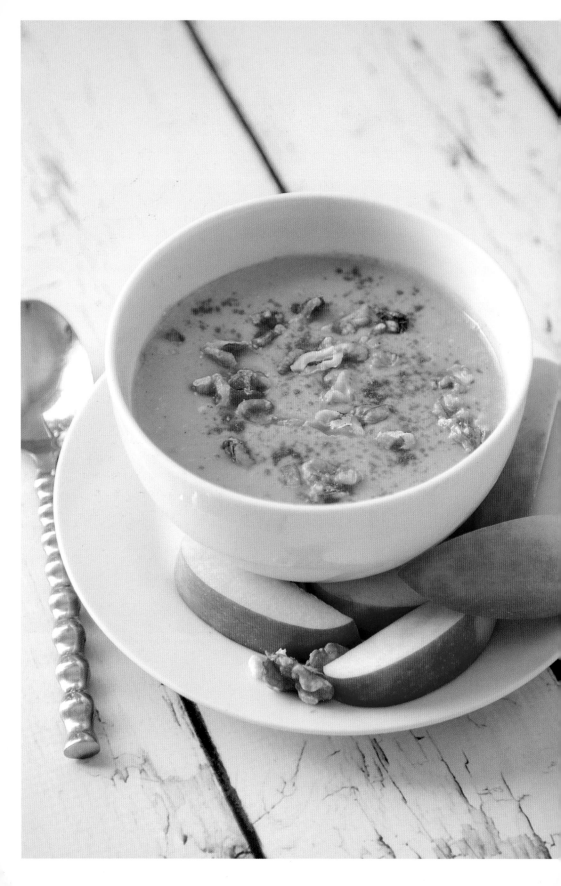

Butternut Squash SOUP

I am a sucker for creamy soups, especially when they involve orange vegetables. You know how I feel about orange vegetables! Except the difference between my beta-carotene overdose days and now is that I don't rely on them for my sole source of carbohydrates. Now I can enjoy squash and sweet potato as a nutritious side dish or soup blend instead of my end-all, be-all carb of the day. The spices in this soup really bring out the deliciousness, and it's a great warming food after a particularly long (and potentially chilly) day.

1 butternut squash, peeled, seeded, and cubed

2 garlic cloves, peeled

2 small shallots, peeled and halved

1 tablespoon (15 ml) olive oil or (14 g) coconut oil

½ of an apple

2 cups (475 ml) water or vegetable broth

½ teaspoon salt

1 tablespoon (7.5 g) chopped walnuts

Pinch of cumin or nutmeg, depending on your preference

Preheat the oven to 400°F (200°C, gas mark 6).

Toss the squash, garlic, and shallots with the olive oil or coconut oil on a greased pan or a lined baking sheet. Roast for about 40 minutes or until golden brown, flipping once or twice.

Let cool for about 15 minutes and then pour the roasted veggies into a blender or food processor along with the apple, water or broth, and salt and blend until smooth. Add more liquid as needed.

Serve with sunflower seeds and a pinch of cumin or nutmeg.

Yield: 2 to 3 servings

"Cream" of Spinach SOUP (VEGAN)

Sometimes good things came from my solely plant-based diet, and one of those things was my learning the vast importance of nourishing my body with fresh, nutrient-rich vegetables. Good, old-fashioned heavy cream might taste delicious, but it has never made my stomach feel very good after I eat it, and there are other foods I enjoy making that I "sacrifice" for more often. Thankfully, you can easily make lighter, plant-based substitutions for cream—in this case, soaked almonds and hearty veggies. It might not be the decadently rich creamed soup of your childhood dreams, but it is a lean, green, mean alternative if you ask me!

1 tablespoon (15 ml) olive oil
   or (14 g) coconut oil, melted
1 clove of garlic
½ cup (50 g) finely chopped scallion
½ cup (60 g) diced celery
1 cup (71 g) diced broccoli
4 cups (950 ml) vegetable broth
2 cups (60 g) firmly packed
   fresh spinach
½ cup (75 g) soaked raw almonds
   (See note.)

Preheat the oven to 350°F (180°C, gas mark 4).

Heat the oil over medium-high heat in a large saucepan. Add the garlic, scallion, celery, and broccoli and sauté until soft and golden brown.

Stir in the vegetable broth and bring to a boil. Reduce the heat to medium and simmer for 10 minutes. Add the spinach and simmer for 10 minutes more or until the leaves are tender.

Stir in the nuts and pour the soup into a blender. Blend on high for 2 minutes or until a thick, creamy consistency is reached.

Serve with salt and pepper, as desired.

Yield: 1 to 2 servings.

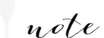

note

To soak the almonds, simply place the raw nuts in a bowl, cover with filtered water, and leave overnight, or for 6 to 8 hours.

Green Goddess RAW SOUP (VEGAN)

How delightfully fresh is a dinner full of raw veggies . . . in a bowl . . . blended together into a soup? That's right . . . *extremely*. Somehow there is something significantly more satisfying about a soup than a salad, even if it has all the same ingredients. Note: Make this soup a few hours in advance if possible to help the flavors meld and to allow the soup to take on a thicker consistency.

1 cup (47 g) romaine lettuce
1 cup (67 g) kale
1 cucumber
4 stalks of celery
1 sliced tomato
1 clove of garlic
1 cup (235 ml) water
¼ cup (4 g) fresh cilantro, optional
1 tablespoon (15 ml) olive oil
2 tablespoons (14 g) ground cumin
Juice of ¼ of a lemon
Salt and pepper, to taste
¼ cup (30 g) chopped walnuts or
    (35 g) pine nuts (or nut of choice)
5 sliced cherry tomatoes

Wash and chop all your vegetables so they can easily blend.

Blend or process the veggies, garlic, water, cilantro, if using, olive oil, cumin, lemon juice, salt, and pepper in a food processor and then pour into a lovely soup bowl. Allow to sit for a few hours, if possible.

Top with walnuts and cherry tomatoes. Ta-da! Enjoy.

Yield: 1 to 2 servings

note

If you're looking at this recipe and worrying that it doesn't seem like the satisfying dinner you are accustomed to, fear not—you can dress it up however you'd like! Serve it on the side of a fresh fish fillet or fill it with quinoa or barley.

GOOEY *Eggplant* MOZZARELLA STACKS

Stacks. Isn't that fun to say? I love the thought of stacking nutritious veggies and ooey, gooey cheese to form a pretty darn healthy "sandwich." It's fun to make and almost laughably easy, considering how beautiful and satisfying this dish turns out to be. This is a dish I love to make when friends and family are coming over, because while it is healthy and nutritious, it also has that luscious melted mozzarella cheese in the middle that has been known to bring more than one person to their knees. I love serving this in bigger portions as an alternative to a lasagna type of dish or on the side of lean meat and/or more veggies.

2 large eggplants
4 teaspoons (20 ml) olive oil
1 large red bell pepper
6 slices of mozzarella cheese
1 cup (30 g) fresh spinach
½ cup (12 g) fresh basil
1 tablespoon (15 ml) balsamic vinegar

Preheat the oven to 450°F (230°C, gas mark 8).

Slice each eggplant into 6 even rounds and discard the thinner ends. You now have 12 rounds. Place them on a baking sheet that's greased or lined with parchment paper. Drizzle each with a bit of olive oil.

Bake for 15 minutes or until the slices are softened. While the eggplant bakes, slice the pepper and mozzarella into 6 even slices. Slice the spinach and basil.

Once the eggplant is soft, take it out of the oven and assemble your stacks. Place the pepper, spinach, basil, and mozzarella on top of one eggplant round and top the stack with a second eggplant round.

Season with salt, if you so desire, and place back in the oven at 250°F (120°C, gas mark ½) until the cheese has melted and the stacks are warm. Drizzle with balsamic vinegar and enjoy.

Yield: 4 servings

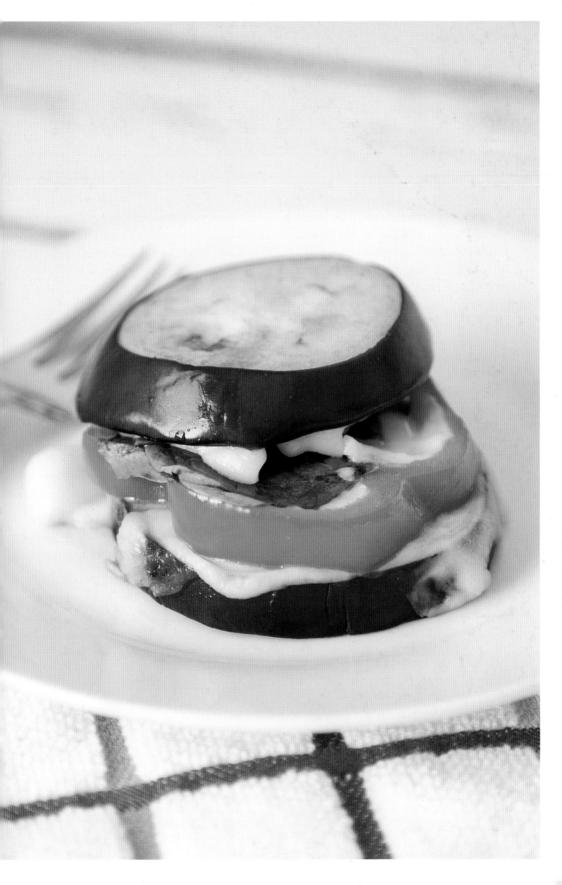

RAW VEGAN *Peanut Butter* CUPS

I eat chocolate like it's my job (ever seen my @chocolateaddicts Instagram account?!), and I can especially clean a plate of chocolate and peanut butter anything. It's no secret that Reese's peanut butter cups are freaking amazing, but they are full of fat, processed milk, and chemical preservatives. Well, thank God I discovered the beauty of raw vegan peanut butter cups because they are my sweet tooth's best friend. This is the number one recipe on my blog, and it was one of the very first I ever shared.

FOR THE FILLING:
½ cup (130 g) natural peanut butter
½ cup (130 g) natural almond butter
1 tablespoon (20 g) agave syrup
2 tablespoons (28 g) organic coconut
   oil, melted

FOR THE CHOCOLATE SHELL:
½ cup (40 g) raw cacao powder
1 tablespoon (20 g) agave syrup
⅓ cup (75 g) coconut oil, melted
¼ cup (44 g) organic dairy-free
   chocolate chips

Grease a muffin or mini-muffin pan with butter or coconut oil or use muffin pan liners.

To make the filling: Combine the nut butters, agave syrup, and coconut oil in a bowl and stir until the ingredients are thoroughly mixed.

Place a spoonful of the mixture into each muffin cup until you have used it all. Place the peanut butter portion in the freezer until hardened. Now it's time to start on the chocolate portion!

To make the chocolate shell: Combine the cacao powder, agave syrup, coconut oil, and chocolate chips in a bowl and stir until thoroughly mixed.

Place a spoonful of the chocolate mixture over the hardened peanut butter mixture.

Pop the peanut butter cups back into the freezer until hardened. Now comes the hard part . . . waiting until they are frozen so you can enjoy!

Yield: 9 to 12 peanut butter cups

note

You can do 1 cup (260 g) of one nut butter or the other, but I love the variety of flavor in using ½ cup (130 g) of each.

You may substitute the agave syrup with maple syrup, honey, or molasses.

PUMPKIN *Almond Butter* OAT BARS

I might be biased because of my intense love for fall and all things pumpkin, but these oat bars are one of my very favorite creations. They can fall into the dessert category because of their sweetness, but they also have enough nutritional value to make the perfect breakfast bar, post-workout refuel, or midday snack. There's nothing I love more than a versatile recipe! And if you want to know a little secret, this raw batter happens to make a perfectly delectable breakfast on its own.

½ cup (130 g) natural almond butter

2 cups (160 g) oats (gluten-free, if necessary)

1 cup (245 g) pumpkin puree

½ cup (160 g) agave syrup (You may substitute with honey, maple syrup, or molasses.)

1 tablespoon (15 ml) vanilla extract

1 teaspoon cinnamon

1 teaspoon baking soda

½ cup (88 g) dairy-free chocolate chips

2 tablespoons (14 g) ground flaxseed

¼ cup (30 g) buckwheat flour, optional

Preheat the oven to 350°F (180°C, gas mark 4).

Combine all of the ingredients in a large mixing bowl and mix until a smooth paste forms.

Press the mixture into a well-greased pan (8-inch x 8-inch [20 cm x 20 cm] is preferable) and bake for 35 minutes or until golden brown.

I top mine with extra chocolate chips for presentation and downright yumminess.

Yield: 8 to 10 bars

note

These bars are delicious right out of the oven, but I also enjoy them refrigerated. They last in the refrigerator for up to a week. (PS: I had a Pumpkin Almond Butter Oat Bar blooper one Christmas and left the mixture sitting out on the counter for about three hours before I put it into the oven . . . they didn't turn out so well! Be forewarned.)

NUTTY *Banana* COOKIES

These cookies are my number-one breakfast-time jam. Munching on one of these with green tea or a glass of warm water with lemon while the sun rises is my version of heaven. Add in a little bit of calming music and a neck massage, and I'm kind of the happiest person on earth. When I was vegan, I made these cookies without the egg all the time, but now I enjoy using the egg for some extra protein, substance, and binding properties. Plus, the combination of bananas, almond butter, and chocolate will simply never get old.

2 eggs

½ cup (56 g) ground flaxseed

½ cup (130 g) almond butter

3 overripe bananas, mashed

2 tablespoons (40 g) agave syrup
   (You may substitute with honey,
   maple syrup, or molasses.)

1 teaspoon pure vanilla extract

½ teaspoon baking soda

⅓ cup (27 g) rolled oats, gluten-free
   if necessary

¼ cup (30 g) crushed walnuts

¼ cup (44 g) dairy-free chocolate chips

Preheat the oven to 350°F (180°C, gas mark 4).

Line a baking sheet with parchment paper and set aside.

Whisk together the eggs, flaxseed, and almond butter until smooth. Add the bananas, agave, vanilla extract, and baking soda and mix thoroughly. Stir in the oats, walnuts, and chocolate chips.

Take a spoonful of the dough, roll it into a ball, and then flatten the top with the back of a spoon or your palm to form a cookie shape. Place on the parchment paper–lined baking sheet.

Repeat that process until the dough is gone, placing the cookies 2 inches (5 cm) apart on the baking sheet.

Bake for about 15 to 20 minutes or until golden brown.

Let the cookies cool for about 20 minutes before enjoying.

Yield: 12 to 14 cookies, depending on the size

FLOURLESS *Chocolate* MUFFINS

These are suitable for any health-conscious foodie *and* any chocolate lover. I am a little bit *too* passionate about combining the two as often as possible, so don't mind me over here whipping up chocolate recipes that are both healthy and decadently delicious. The fact that these are flourless means they are naturally gluten-free, and they get their sweetness from the natural sources of banana and honey. And don't skimp on the chocolate chips—everyone likes a good chunky, chippy bite here and there!

1 large overripe banana

1 large egg

½ cup (130 g) peanut butter

⅓ cup (27 g) natural cocoa powder or raw cacao powder

3 tablespoons (60 g) honey (You may substitute with agave syrup, brown rice syrup, or maple syrup.)

1 tablespoon (15 ml) pure vanilla extract

½ teaspoon baking soda

½ cup (88 g) mini semisweet chocolate chips, dairy-free optional

Preheat the oven to 350°F (180°C, gas mark 4).

In a blender or food processor, combine all the ingredients except for the chocolate chips. You will have to stop and scrape the sides a few times. (And taste the batter while you're at it because it's kind of heavenly and amazing.)

Once blended, spoon the batter into lined muffin tins. The batter is sticky, so you will probably need to lick your fingers. (Or be really, really diligent with the spoon.)

Sprinkle the chocolate chips on top of each muffin. Place in the oven and bake for 15 to 20 minutes or until the edges are golden brown.

Let them cool before you enjoy. Store them in the fridge for up to a week! You can also freeze them for longer storage.

Yield: 12 muffins

HEALTHY *Banana* SPLIT

I think it goes without saying that banana splits are one of the most delicious desserts out there. And if you really think about it, they do stem from a semblance of healthiness. We have the banana—score, both delicious and packed full of nutrients—and the nuts, full of protein and healthy fats, and the rest is kind of left up to us to figure it out. By substituting a healthier alternative for the traditional ice cream, chocolate sauce, and processed toppings, we can make a sweet and satisfying dessert that also gives us energy and makes us feel great afterward.

¼ cup (20 g) raw cacao powder

4 tablespoons (56 g) coconut oil, melted

2 tablespoons (40 g) honey
(You may substitute with agave syrup, maple syrup, or molasses.)

1 cup (230 g) Greek yogurt or dairy-free Greek-style yogurt

1 medium banana, sliced

½ cup (85 g) sliced strawberries

2 tablespoons (22 g) mini semisweet chocolate chips or dairy-free chocolate chips

¼ cup (28 g) slivered almonds

Combine the cacao powder, coconut oil, and honey in a small bowl and stir thoroughly. Place in the fridge and allow to sit and thicken for a few minutes.

Pour the yogurt into a bowl and top with banana, strawberries, slivered almonds, and chocolate chips.

Once the raw chocolate sauce has thickened, pour it over the yogurt bowl and enjoy.

GLUTEN-FREE *Apple* TARTLET

While my mom and I have always been chocolate fans whenever it comes to choosing a dessert, my dad has been the fruit pie type of guy. An apple tart is usually his very favorite go-to. When I ditched the processed foods lifestyle, I went on a mission to create the perfect healthy apple tart for my dad that he would not only *pretend to kind of like* (and then let it sit on the counter for a week and get old), but that he would actually *enjoy*! After much trial and error, this recipe finally did the trick. This one's for you, Daddio!

FOR THE CRUST:

1½ cups (168 g) almond flour (or any other gluten-free flour of choice)
½ cup (72 g) coconut sugar
⅓ cup (43 g) cornstarch
8 tablespoons (112 g) grass-fed butter or ghee
1 large egg
1 tablespoon (15 ml) pure vanilla extract

FOR THE FILLING:

6 medium apples, peeled, cored, and thinly sliced
½ cup (72 g) coconut sugar
1 tablespoon (7 g) cinnamon
½ tablespoon (4 g) nutmeg
¼ teaspoon sea salt

FOR THE CRUMBLE:

½ cup (72 g) coconut sugar
¼ cup (28 g) almond flour (See same substitution as above.)
½ tablespoon (4 g) cinnamon
¼ cup (55 g) grass-fed butter or ghee

Preheat the oven to 400°F (200°C, gas mark 6).

To make the crust: In a mixing bowl, stir together all of the crust ingredients until well combined. Knead it with your hands until the consistency feels thick and solid. Divide it into 2 pieces, putting one half in the refrigerator and one half in the freezer.

After 20 minutes, remove the refrigerated dough and roll it out to the thickness of your desired pie crust. Place the crust in a greased glass pie dish and use a fork to poke holes evenly in the sides and bottom.

To make the filling: Combine all the filling ingredients. Pour over the dough in the baking dish.

To make the crumble: Mix together all of the ingredients. Use a fork or a handheld mixer on low speed to break up the butter or ghee if need be. Make sure the mixture remains crumbly and doesn't get too smooth.

Sprinkle the crumble topping over the apple filling until it is evenly distributed on top of the pie. Use aluminum foil to cover the edges of the crust to make sure it doesn't burn.

Bake for 35 to 40 minutes or until the topping is lightly browned and the filling is starting to bubble. Let the pie cool for at least an hour before serving.

Yield: 12 servings

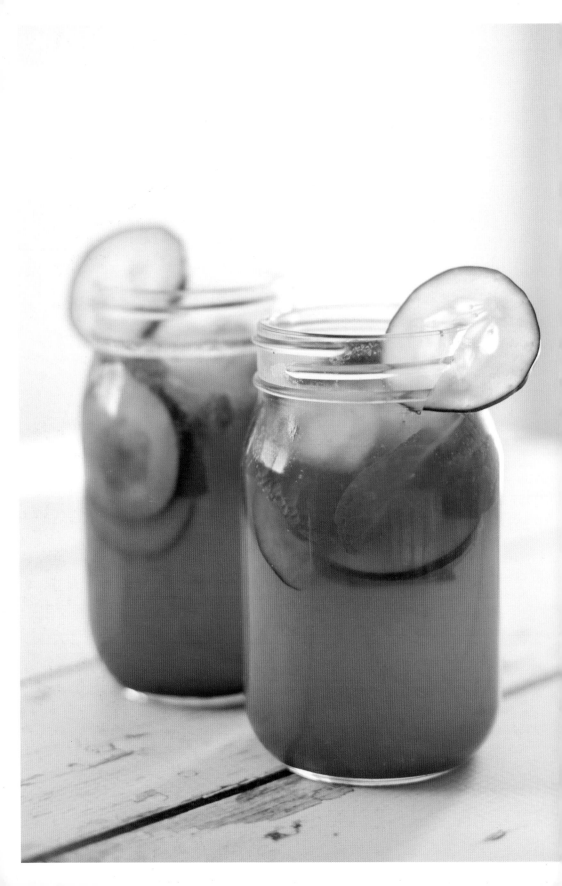

SPARKLING *Lime* CUCUMBERADE

This is my personal favorite drink to sip on when I'm out or when I have friends over, with or without vodka. It's light and refreshing with a rosy hue from the coconut sugar, and it gives you that tangy zing from the lime with the freshness of the cucumber. I have always been a fan of cucumber water, and for this reason I think my Cucumberade is fit for a spa day. If you're into that idea, blast some spa music while you whip this baby up, put on a bathrobe and your favorite face mask, and sip away.

¼ cup (30 g) coconut sugar

1 tablespoon (6 g) lime zest

1 cup (235 ml) water

¼ cup (24 g) fresh mint leaves

1 cup (235 ml) lime juice

1 medium cucumber, halved
and thinly sliced

2 cups (475 ml) sparkling water

Combine the coconut sugar, lime zest, and water in a saucepan over medium-high heat. Bring to a simmer and stir constantly until the sugar has dissolved. Remove from the heat and stir in the mint leaves. Let it sit for 25 to 30 minutes.

Strain your homemade lime syrup through a mesh sieve. Combine it with the lime juice and cucumber. Refrigerate for at least 1 hour.

To serve, add in the sparkling water and optional vodka. Serve over ice. Enjoy!

Yield: 2 servings

note

If you're more into the idea of making this as a cocktail to enjoy with friends, add a few shots of vodka and you're golden. You'll hardly be able to taste it.

CIDER SPRITZER

This drink takes me way back to my apple-picking, hay-barreling, denim-outfit-wearing (yes, I mean entire outfits made of denim) days growing up in Northern California. It is so distinctly fall with its warming cinnamon and grated fresh ginger, but you can make it at any time of year! You get bonus points for drinking it alongside a slice of pumpkin pie!

2 cups (475 ml) apple cider

1 cinnamon stick

1 orange, halved and squeezed

1 knob of grated fresh ginger

1 cup (235 ml) sparkling water

Combine the apple cider, cinnamon, the orange and its skin, and the grated ginger in a saucepan over medium-high heat. Boil for 10 to 15 minutes.

Strain the mixture into a glass or jar and let it cool.

To serve, add in the sparkling water and serve over ice. Enjoy!

Yield: 2 servings

GINGER MOJITO MOCKTAIL

Okay, yum. I am a sucker for anything with ginger in it, but the fact that this drink boasts the delish combo of ginger, mint, *and* lime just throws me over the edge a little bit. This drink is super versatile because not only is it a great summertime poolside drink, but it's equally appropriate for the holidays, a date night, or a brunch with girlfriends. If you'd like to add gin or vodka, be my guest! I told you it was versatile.

8 fresh mint leaves

2 ounces (60 ml) fresh lime juice

4 teaspoons (27 g) honey or
   (12 g) coconut sugar

1 knob of grated fresh ginger

2 cups (475 ml) sparkling water

In a tall glass, muddle the mint leaves and lime juice. You can do this with a traditional drink muddler or the back end of a fork.

Add the honey or coconut sugar and the ginger. Stir until combined thoroughly. Fill the glass with ice cubes.

Pour in sparkling water and optional gin or vodka. Enjoy!

Yield: 2 servings

17

THE BALANCED WRAP-UP

**Health and happiness are not simply a matter of eating well, looking
your best, and being clean and pure. Sometimes being healthy and
happy requires getting messy, by looking inward and dealing with the
chaotic jumble of truths that come up. In my eating disorder recovery
and my transition from the strictest plant-based lifestyle you can imagine, I came to find that the best things in life came from stepping
outside of my comfort zone and allowing things to be. Let me tell you,
that's a crazy thought for someone whose entire life was regimented by
green-juice-to-exercise ratio for so long.**

Being healthy and happy is much more a matter of balance than anything
else. Eat your greens, but eat that cupcake when you want it! When you allow
yourself to eat whatever your body craves in a mindful way, it doesn't become
such an obsessive phenomenon anymore. It just becomes a part of life—and
that's exactly what food should be. It should fuel us, and we should enjoy
every ounce of it! And then we should move on with our day and squeeze the
most out of it that we possibly can.

Balance is an ebb and flow. Some days, I feel like I have everything in
check, and life feels balanced and superbly manageable. Other days, finding
my balance is harder to work toward, but I don't give up on it. And I certainly
don't obsess over it. Or at least I try not to! Instead I forgive myself, and I
remember I'm human. Being human is a lot more fun than that superhuman
willpower I used to spend so much time and effort trying to maintain.

And, if you ever feel lost or in a rut or totally off-kilter and not balanced, take
a deep breath, be kind to yourself, and remember that it's going to be okay.
If all else fails, head over to TheBalancedBlonde.com, click on the contact
form, and pour your heart out. I just poured my heart out to you, after all.

Lots of love, forever & always,
Jordan Younger // *The Balanced Blonde*

ACKNOWLEDGMENTS

It's very important for me to acknowledge everyone who has played a role in bringing this book to life because along the way not only did book-related things go down, but an extremely personal recovery journey along with it. I am grateful for each and every one of you.

Sarah Passick, otherwise known as the Jesse Pinkman to my Walter White. Thank you for believing in this book before it even existed. Thank you for being my greatest advocate, my cheerleader, my words of wisdom, and my friend. *Breaking Vegan* would still be hanging out in my brain if it weren't for our collaborative vision and your expertise. Thank you.

Amanda Waddell, another extremely instrumental figure in giving this book life. You believed in this story before I could even put it into words, and you showed me patience when I needed it most. Your guidance, editing, and friendship have been invaluable.

To everyone at Fair Winds Press, from the marketing dream team to the editing powerhouses to the talented art department—Heather, Cara, Kathy, Katie, Becky, Lisa, Winnie, and everyone at the publishing company who helped along the way. Thank you.

Tynan Daniels, for your vision, your talent, and your unbelievable dedication to helping me bring my creative dreams to life on a daily basis. Thank you for capturing the cover of this book, for being my right-hand man, and above all for your friendship and kind heart. I am so lucky to have you in my life.

To the readers of *The Balanced Blonde*, both new and longstanding, thank you. If you had told me when I started my blog in June 2013 that I would develop a community of incredible, beautiful, shining souls who have become my friends from all over the world, I wouldn't have believed I could ever be so lucky. Without your support, I would be nowhere near where I am today. I love you all immeasurably.

To my small but mighty TBB Team, thank you for believing in me, for helping me make my brand what it is, and for continuing to build with me. Ali, Cyrus, and Morgan, I wouldn't be here without you.

My dear friends, my soulmates. You know who you are! Thank you for showing me love and understanding, even when I was so caught up in my strict vegan lifestyle that I probably didn't eat with you for many months. And thank you for going to obscure restaurants with me throughout. But above all, thank you for your endless support and for being a part of this process.

Katie Estep, thank you for being my lifelong everything and for being incredible before, during, and after this whole process—and always. Jillian Jaime, for reminding me that enjoyment comes first and for your extremely dear friendship in my life. Danielle Kesich, for the endless support and for having my back no matter how crazy the crazies got. Tommy Genovese, for understanding me inside out and then some. Isabella Renee, for being the other half of my heart. Paul Florez, for being my writing partner and dear friend and believing in me always. Tara Milhem, for every ounce of truth and meaning you've brought to my life.

Steven Bratman, for your brilliance and for guiding me toward recovery by simply inventing the term I was suffering from. I am forever grateful for you. Lauren LaMay and Brooke Wells, for helping me fall in love with writing, and for always believing in me.

Hugely, my family. You have shown me kindness, love, and support in following my dreams in every way, and that will never be lost on me. Mama, you are my best friend and there are no words. Daddy, my respect and love for you go beyond this universe. All of my siblings and my beautiful nieces and nephew, thank you for always being there. Jojo loves you.

Last but not least, to the beautiful and strong community of individuals suffering from eating disorders of all kinds. You are not alone. You are heard. You've got this.

ABOUT THE AUTHOR

Jordan Younger is a health and lifestyle blogger living in sunny Los Angeles, California. She is passionate about bringing health and happiness to as many people as possible through her blog, *The Balanced Blonde*, her popular YouTube channel, and her various forms of social media. Jordan has a health-inspired clothing line, TBV Apparel, and a line of health-related mobile apps with content from recipes to restaurant reviews. She has appeared on *Good Morning America*, *Nightline*, *CBS News*, *Larry King Now*, *NPR*, and more sharing her health journey and recovery story. This is her first book and her most cherished project to date.

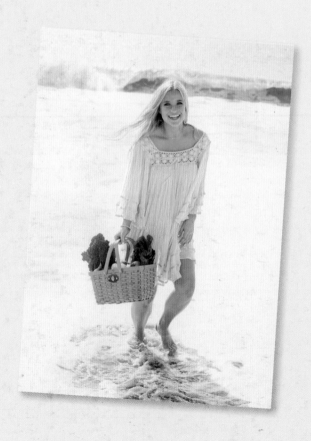